LIFE SUPPORT

THE HEALING POWER OF THE STAPLES

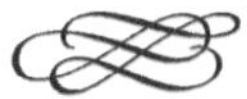

SHALAMANTU WISDOM

CONTENTS

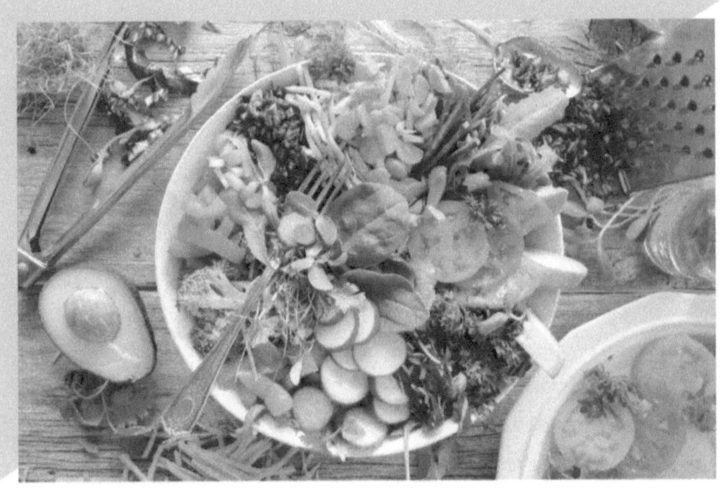

The Superfoods Checklist

Foods that Superhumans are made of

This checklist includes:
- Foods that help with brain function
- Cures for viral infections
- Vegetables that help manage stress
- Spices that improve skin health
- And much, much, much more!

This list should be the first part of
everyone's grocery list to transform your
health and your life.

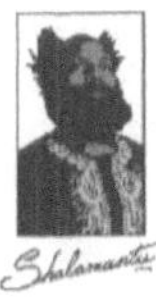

To receive this life changing tool, scan the QR Code or visit the link
www.shalamantu.com/lifeupgrade

"As we begin to pass less harsh judgement on others, we can begin to look at ourselves with less angst, guilt and severe judgement. This will lead to acceptance of ourselves and our communities. The result of more understanding is more wise decisions being made. I have always believed that tolerance turns to acceptance, and acceptance can lead to rejoicing in the differences that we share. This does not mean turning a blind eye to injustice or malicious behaviours. But seeing another person struggle by doing ill will to others will give a person strength and understanding in the midst of life turbulence. When we realize that each of us has a long way to go to become the person of our dreams, we can look with a different heart at those whose actions we do not understand yet. And we can attempt to treat them and ourselves as people who are doing our best at this moment to get to a higher path, regardless of how off-course from that trail we may be."

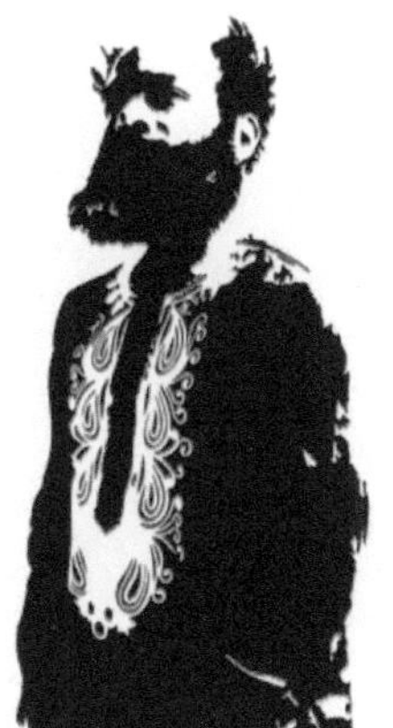

INTRODUCTION

We are living in disturbing times in which diseases, obesity, pollution, and mental health issues are the norm. How did we get here? What did people in olden times do differently? In spite of the growing mountains of information on healthy living and foods, the world seems lost. What is healthy today becomes unhealthy tomorrow. Diets have changed over time, from wild animals and grains to highly processed foodstuffs. Interestingly, diseases have increased and evolved, as well.

Carbohydrates have acquired a terrible reputation as unhealthy and fattening foods over the years. There is general confusion on the role of carbohydrates in our diets and whether to consume or eliminate them. The lack of credible information on the pros and cons of eating carbohydrates does not help much. At some point, most of us have wondered whether to take in carbohydrates or not for better health and a great body. In fact, at any given time, nearly half of people are on a diet for weight loss, weight gain, or better health. The others have either just completed a diet or given up and embarked on a binge. Carbohydrates remain the biggest victims of diets, labeled as bad foods and the first to go from the plate. Yet, they have been staple foods for many generations of people.

The search for answers in healthy lifestyles and environmental stewardship is on, and *Life Support* is here to provide some of these answers. In this book, we will look at carbohydrates, humanity's staples of the past and present, as well as the pros and cons of their consumption. The book also provides information on whether you should add them to your diet or eliminate them. Moreover, it looks at how these foods have affected our health over the years as well as aided in sustaining civilization. With this knowledge available, you will be in a position to consume carbohydrates in a manner that boosts your health. Not only is this book educative, but also crucial in aiding healthy weight loss, promoting environmental consciousness, and ensuring a healthy lifestyle.

That is not all. Read on to learn how different people across the world, past and present, prepare their staple foods. Here is an opportunity to improve your creativity in the kitchen and awaken your adventurous spirit. Explore different staple foods and decide what to add to your diet. Learn the effects of different foods on both personal and social well being. As a bonus, the information in this resource will improve your social life by enabling you to converse confidently on matters of food and earn the respect of your social circle.

You can be sure that at the end of this book, you will be in a position to make an informed choice on what to include in your diet. Considering that what you eat affects your outlook, health, and state of mind, this information is life-changing. Do not wonder what to eat anymore, put aside those fears you have carried over the years, and claim a life full of health and happiness, and an attractive body to hold it all.

Why waste more time on top of all those years? Let's get started.

CHAPTER ONE: OUT OF THE COLD

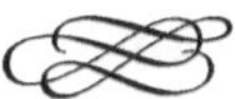

A LONG TIME AGO

Our ancestors gathered and scavenged for food. Anthropologists around the globe have spent a lot of time and research into the diets of our ancestors. The main focus of their work is on the Old Stone Age, also referred to as the Paleolithic. If you have heard of the Paleo Diet, you now know its origin. The Old Stone Age was a prehistoric period of about 2.5 million years ago in which early man developed and used stone tools. In this age, we had some relatives, the Neanderthals and the Denisovans, who are now sadly extinct. Typically, the period was divided into three parts: the Lower, Middle, and Upper Paleolithic. In those ancient days, the earth was considerably colder, with glacial expansions. Humans, therefore, lived in groups and were nomads. They hunted large mammals such as deer, woolly mammoths, and giant bison for food. Using stone tools, they cut, crushed, and pounded meat to ease the absorption of nutrients. Fire was yet to be invented in the early part of the Stone Age, so humans consumed food in its raw state. If you enjoy your steak rare, thank your ancestors.

Roughly 14,000 years ago, it is thought that global warming began, although not at the current rate. The warming of the earth caused the extinction of most of the large Ice Age animals due to an unfavorable environment. On the other hand, warmth favored the growth of barley and wheat. The consumption of these increased, prompting humans to begin settling down. The nomadic lifestyles of the Ice Age dwindled and semi-permanent housing emerged. Humans were now out of the cold.

THE END OF HUNTING AND GATHERING

Being out of the cold did not mean that we were civilized and no longer hunted and gathered. On the contrary, without the need to move around much, humans had time to explore and develop an intricate knowledge of both animal and plant life. Equipped with better tools and fire, our human ancestors did not scavenge, but rather killed animals for food. They also devised ways of storing food for later use. Hunting and gathering were a way of life not only for Homo heidelbergensis, who lived between 700,000 and 200,000 years ago, but also for Homo sapiens.

CHAPTER SUMMARY

The most important points to pick from this chapter include the facts that the environment has always provided for us: that carbohydrates, mainly cereals, were the first crops to be domesticated, and that ancient man thrived on cereals such as wheat, barley, and pulses.

In the next chapter, you will learn how agriculture changed our lives, making them easier or more complicated, depending on your point of view. Leaving behind the hunting and gathering way of life contributed to civilization, allowing us to specialize in other areas of life.

CHAPTER TWO: HOW DID THIS CHANGE US?

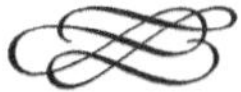

Many of us today cannot imagine life without domestic animals and plants. As a matter of fact, there are some of us who cannot even begin to understand the life of foraging for plants and setting traps for animals. We now live in an industrialized world, where food comes from stores that get it from factories. We have limited interaction with actual animals and plants. Life, as you know it, and the ease of getting food to your plate, is all thanks to the domestication of plants and animals.

While most of the focus is on the domestication of plants, animals also played a crucial role. I find it offensive to them to relegate them to the side without due acknowledgment. Besides being a more reliable source of food, animals worked the land in preparation for planting, were involved in weeding, and provided manure to enrich the land. The success of crop farming relied much on animals. Additionally, animals such as the dog provided security that enabled man to undertake the domestication of other animals and crops without fear of attacks from wild predators.

The success of the domestication process changed the human way of life and is considered one of the most meaningful advancements in humanity's history. With the population able to have adequate food from a few people, there was no need to spend the entire day looking for food. We now breathe easy knowing that we have certain control over how much food we produce and when. Technological advancement and the honing of farming skills ensured that we grow crops throughout the year. Growing our own food kept us in permanent homes. While previously people had settled for a while before moving when need occurred, the production of food saw the development of permanent housing. Villages developed, and so did cities. The earliest villages and cities in the world were built in agricultural areas, near fields of crops.

With a sense of permanence and food, humans explored ways of cultivating a wide variety of seeds and breeding animals. The number of cultivated crops grew substantially over the years. Among these, corn, rice, and wheat are the most popular in the world. The concentration on farming also led to increased food supplies, prompting the need for proper storage. Consequently, the population increased with success in growing and storing food, creating a need for more food and providing the labor to do so. Trade grew as a result of surplus food and cities developed.

DID IT MAKE OUR LIVES EASIER?

We can all attest that having adequate food is one of the best things in life. If we were all guaranteed a meal each day, some people would not bother to work. Fortunately or unfortunately, life does not work that way. Food comes from sweat. Some may argue that it was better in the olden days, when all you needed to do is wander into the forest and come back with fruit and nuts. They're probably right, but life wasn't easy then, either. Hunting and gathering food required skills and the ability to fight off other hungry animals. Imagine the pain of getting honey in those days. In addition to bee stings, you would have to ward off raccoons, honey badgers, and bears. But growing our crops is not easy, either. Farmers put in long hours of hard labor and have to worry about the weather and diseases.

Some of the responsibilities and bills you have are an indirect result of agriculture. Without cultivating crops and keeping animals, we would still be hunting, gathering, and moving around. Lovers of the environment would rejoice at the preservation of nature. There would be no pollution from pesticides or food manufacturing plants. Desertification would be a foreign concept, and the world would most likely be green. You would not even need to pay your mortgage, water bill, or electric bill. The city you live in today is there because our ancestors domesticated crops and animals. You would not even need to pay tuition fees, as there would be no formal school, only the jungle school. Do you think this would be a better life?

Well, before you curse your ancestors, remember you most likely would not have been born if there were no adequate food production. If you were lucky enough to be part of the world, your diet would only consist of foods available in your locality. There would be no formal government, organized religion, or education, as we have today. Agriculture led to the development of cities, which caused the need for governments, brought about organized religion and trade, and opened up the world.

You have a career and friends across the world due to the domestication of plants and animals. Otherwise, you would be out there looking for food. Besides, there is a deliberate promotion of sustainable agricultural methods that protect ecological systems and offset climatic challenges. Such methods ensure food diversity by the growth of environment-tolerant crops and preservation of water. In the recent past, there has been an increased emphasis on organic agriculture due to the growing awareness of the harm caused by conventional methods of farming. Farmers are shying away from the use of unnecessary fertilizers and pesticides. Instead, they use organic methods like crop rotation, use of cover crops, and mulching.

Yes, agriculture does make our life easier. There is adequate food supply to meet our needs and support the growing human population. In a bid to reach the consumer, farmers' markets have opened across the world to provide fresh products without long distribution chains. Furthermore, the mass production of food has further necessitated value addition. Local stores stock up items such as tomato paste, yogurt, pastries, and pasta, making access easy. We no longer have to labor to refine seeds into food items that we want or take time to process anything. Food is available in whatever form one desires. Today we even have pre-cooked food in the stores for busy people. Consequently, we have time to travel, work, learn, and even worry about our weight. Agriculture has literally given us the freedom to become what we desire and do as we please.

WHAT FREEDOM?

Food is a basic need, alongside shelter and clothing. However, not everyone is food-secure. According to the Food and Agriculture Organization (FAO), over 820 million people lack enough to eat. Paradoxically, overweight and obesity rates are on the rise. The good news is that the majority of people have the freedom to eat what they want and when they want. There are all kinds of foods available to choose from. Advances in transport and communication have facilitated the movement of all types of food around the globe. You can have sushi in America and pizza in Japan. The rich variety of food serves all our needs: energy, medicinal value, comfort, or budget.

The agriculture and food industries are worth over $8 trillion. FAO reports that more than one billion people, or one in three workers, get their income from agriculture. Over 60 percent of the entire workforce in sub-Saharan Africa works in this sector. Therefore, agriculture puts money directly into the pockets of over a billion people, who then purchase other services and products. In essence, if the agriculture and food industry were to shut down today, global economies would come tumbling down.

If you think that money does not come into your pocket, consider your profession. The earliest manufacturing industries were food-driven. Plant domestication caused advancements in tool production. From the initial stone tools of the stone age to metal tools used in the bronze age, humans realized the need for efficient tools to drive food production. From simple hand-digging tools, plows that used animal power were invented. Thus began the Industrial Revolution. The Agricultural Revolution of the mid-eighteenth century was a result of the difficulty associated with agricultural work. People had to innovate and invent to ease the labor, which in turn laid the foundation for the Industrial Revolution. The innovations and inventions made work less labor-intensive, freeing workers to industrial jobs. Thus, the domestication of plants and animals propelled the Industrial Revolution. The ease of movement and communication we enjoy today stemmed from agriculture.

As earlier stated, the emergence of permanent human settlements was due to agriculture. Population centers and cities developed in agricultural areas before spreading to other areas. The cities had to find a way to administer and tax people. Formal governments thus began stimulating the beginning of writing, which in turn played a crucial role in the transformation of societies into civilizations.

The world population has increased considerably over the years. In the days of hunting and gathering, the human population was estimated at 6-10 million people, which was the earth's capacity. Now there are about 7.7 billion people, thanks to food production. All these people depend on roughly 570 million farms for food. With adequate food and time, people have been able to focus and specialize in other economic activities, like the manufacturing of different products and trade. Specialization is a proven way of increasing productivity, which has caused civilization to grow by leaps and bounds.

Since we do not need to forage for food and farmers are feeding us, we have time to communicate, travel, learn other skills, and enjoy life. The availability of food to the masses is an enabling factor for socialization and a key factor in politics. In essence, we can now live full lives due to agricultural production.

EFFECT OF PLANT AND ANIMAL DOMESTICATION ON PEOPLE LIVING IN COLD CLIMATES

Early humans lived in cold climates, particularly during the Ice Age. Climatic adaptation, which is a species' genetic adaptation to environmental conditions, came into play. Their physique evolved into short and wide bodies suitable for heat conservation. Diet played a key role in their survival hence they relied on raw meat, as well as cooked food. Previously, humans avoided living in cold environments due to the challenges of foraging in a harsh environment. In extreme cold, there were few crops available, since the ground was mostly covered by frost. Most animals hibernated, significantly limiting available food over the winter. Thus, finding food in such places was difficult. People, therefore, opted to move to warmer climates, where food was accessible throughout the year.

The domestication of plants and animals opened up the world so people could comfortably survive in colder climates. By growing crops in those areas, the people were certain about the availability of food even in the harshest of weather. Some of the crops that have been grown in cold climates include potatoes, peas, and a wide variety of vegetables, such as carrots, turnips, and beets. In Turkey, for example, people use the cold climate to grow cereals, such as wheat and barley.

With the ability to produce adequate foods, humans were able to thrive in cold climates. They further domesticated animals, such as cattle, llamas, pigs, sheep, and goats. As such, despite the cold, they could get milk, meat, and crops. Life in cold climates, therefore, became bearable, particularly with man's ability to grow and store feeds for use when the weather is too harsh. Today, humans inhabit all parts of the world, as they are assured of the food supply.

ADDITIONAL SOURCES OF ENERGY

Despite shifting away from hunting and gathering as a way of life and domesticating plants and animals for food, humans had to ensure the consumption of foods that increased energy levels. The need for more energy was further necessitated by the farming that required intensive labor. In addition to the crops grown at home, humans had to find other complementary sources of food to boost energy levels.

One of those complementary foods is meat. Our ancestors initially scavenged for meat before acquiring skills to hunt both small and large animals. Scientists think that meat intake may have played a crucial role in the evolution of humans' larger brains. The intake of calorie-dense meat and bone marrow by Homo erectus, in particular, helped to fuel his brain. A higher-quality bulky plant fiber diet could have resulted in smaller guts for humans, but the energy from the food could have been easily used up by the brain. Our brains are greedy, taking up approximately 20 percent of our energy during rest. To date, meat forms a part of our diet and is usually paired with cereal products, such as wheat, corn, and other grains.

Despite the domestication of animals and plants, humans suffered from some food-related illnesses, mainly from eating the same variety of grains each day. With time, their health was affected, despite having animals for meat and milk, since those animals also came with pests and diseases. At other times, there was no meat to go with the cereals. In those moments, the women came in handy as the foragers. Yes, foraging continued, albeit at a low rate, for calorie-rich foods, like nuts, yams, chestnuts, and tubers. The Australian original peoples, for example, rely on water chestnuts and nutgrass to provide additional energy. Similarly, humans today eat a variety of nuts and tubers to increase energy levels.

Fatty fish have been part of the human diet since the Paleolithic Age. The Inuit people in the Arctic traditionally obtained almost all their calories from fish, seals, and narwhals. Fish not only provides proteins and fatty acids but also vitamin B_{12}, which works with folic acid to aid the production of red blood cells. Having optimal red blood cells increases energy levels and reduces fatigue. Humans consume a variety of fish in their diet alongside domesticated crops.

Over time, humans have learned the importance of including a variety of foods in their diet to increase energy levels and obtain nutrients. Eggs have, over the years, become a cheap, stable, and nutritious food. In addition to their ability to satisfy, eggs provide fuel for the body. Their high protein content provides a steady energy source without spiking blood sugar. Eggs are also rich in Vitamin B, which helps enzymes efficiently facilitate food breakdown. Moreover, they have leucine, which stimulates the production of energy by causing fat breakdown and cells' uptake of blood sugar. What makes eggs a good addition to the human diet is their availability at an affordable price in most parts of the world. On average, organic eggs cost between $4 and $7 a dozen while non-organic eggs cost between $0.97 and $3. They are, therefore, commonly found in many households and widely consumed.

Water is life. Our bodies are literally made of 60 percent water, with the heart and brain composed of 73 percent water, lungs 83 percent, skin 64 percent, and kidneys and muscles 79 percent. Water is found within our cells, playing a role in many cellular functions, such as energy production. It is rehydrating, giving the body a refreshing feeling, aiding digestion, boosting energy, and reducing fatigue. Water has been an integral part of the human diet since time immemorial. Without it, the body cannot function efficiently, leading to headaches, grumpiness, physical and mental deterioration. In fact, humans cannot survive more than a week without water. Some scientists claim it only takes 3-4 days of dehydration before a person dies. The importance of water cannot be overstated. Even without food, humans can survive for weeks as long as they consume water. Take your glass and keep rehydrating even when not thirsty. Your body will thank you.

CHAPTER SUMMARY

The domestication of plants and animals brought about change in our way of life by allowing us to participate in other areas of life besides searching for food. Settlements emerged and cities grew, opening up the world to be as it is today. In particular, grains, roots, and tubers are the main carbohydrates that give us energy but they can be supplemented with nuts, fish, and eggs. Include them on your plate. Also, they all work well with water - it is life, so keep rehydrating.

In the next chapter, you will learn the dominant role played by the staple foods in war and sustaining civilization.

CHAPTER THREE: THE ROLE OF STAPLE FOODS IN WAR AND CIVILIZATION

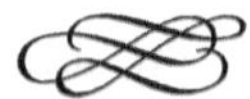

Image source: quoteideas.com

*H*umanity survives on food. With the exception of air and water, food is the most important factor holding life together. If you look closely at the lives of the desert people, you can see that even water can be obtained from food. Ironically, we live in times when we are all either trying to eat less or eat more. The FAO estimates that globally, over 820 million people lack adequate food. On the other hand, the World Health Organization (WHO) reported that by 2016, an excess of 1.9 billion adults were overweight, with more than 650 million being obese. If our ancestors saw these figures, they would consider going back in time and allowing all of us to forage. The walks through the forests and the wild diet would do us a world of good.

The current situation is a clear indication of the place of food in society. Of course, the kinds of foods have changed over time. In ancient times, humans ate natural foods, particularly grains picked from plants and meat from wild animals. The discovery of fire enabled man to cook a wide variety of foods. After the early domestication of plants and animals, diets grew less varied since not all species could be tamed or grown. However, as our brains grew, we began processing food. For example, grains were made into flour before being further made into bread. Over the years, we have taken processing to a much higher level, adding nutrients and flavor to almost all foods. Despite all our technological advancements, grains remain the staple food for most people in the world. Staple foods are routinely consumed in dominant quantities by a majority of the people and contribute to the energy needs of the population. Cereal grains and tubers such as wheat, maize, potatoes, rice, sweet potatoes, cassava, and soybeans are the most common staple foods consumed around the planet.

Throughout history and up to today, food has provided us with the necessary energy for growth and engaging in other undertakings. Without it, all other aspects of life are compromised. The production of food, therefore, is the foundation for all other human's economic and social activities. If you have doubts, walk with me through the process of civilization.

AGRICULTURE AND THE PILLARS OF CIVILIZATION

By now, you know that plant and animal domestication defined life as we know it. As humans and their environment evolved, civilization arose. However, to determine what constitutes civilization, historians identified some essential characteristics of civilized societies. The six most essential ones are cities, government, religion, social structure, writing, and art. For all of them, agriculture played a vital part in their being and continuity.

As earlier discussed, the first permanent settlements were as a result of plant and animal domestication. The ancient civilizations developed around farm areas, particularly in river valleys. The environment in such places was conducive for the large-scale farming needed to feed the large populations. The successful production of food in such quantities that there was surplus catalyzed the development of cities. People from neighboring areas moved to the cities to work, trade, and live. For the first time, strangers lived, worked, and socialized within the same space.

With the convergence of people in cities and no formal administration, a challenge on the effective organization and regulation of human activities arose. Furthermore, due to the increasing number of people coming to the cities, there was a need to maintain a steady supply of food and ensure security. Governments were formed to facilitate relations among people. The previously small and separate communities came together, contributing to the establishment of states that operated under a single administrative structure. The governments were supported by surplus grain taken as tax.

People now lived harmoniously in cities under a formal government structure, but required a unifying cause. So ancient people applied religion in all aspects of life, and religion became a strong unifying factor in early civilizations. Shared beliefs, behaviors, and thoughts on the meaning of life enabled strangers to find common ground, respect each other, and build mutual trust. If you have interacted with strongly religious people, then you know that their spirit of brotherhood overlooks all other differences. Religion eased relations and promoted peace that, in turn, facilitated food production and trade. Furthermore, the firm belief in the supernatural powers of the gods instigated deep respect for the forces of natures as well as an understanding of their roles. People therefore sacrificed and pleased the gods and goddesses for the community's success, including bumper harvests. Moreover, owing to the close relationship between politics and religion, spiritual leaders were influential. In some cases, the same people acted as both religious and political leaders. For instance, in ancient Egypt, the pharaohs were considered as divine kings: either human incarnations or representatives of the gods. Even in cases where the temporal and spiritual powers were different, they worked jointly. The spiritual leaders supported their political counterparts.

Agriculture gave cities adequate food, which gave rise to trade, which gave rise to money. With money came power and class. Further, the religious and political organizations triggered the creation and fortification of social hierarchies. Like today, politicians and religious leaders were at the top of the ladder while the working class, that is, farmers, artisans, and traders, were the middle class. Slaves and unspecialized workers took the bottom shelf. Interestingly, it was these low-class people that did the bulk of the work in food production.

Early civilizations had become sophisticated, which created the need to keep records. The Mesopotamians were the first to invent writing and using it to keep track of transactions, particularly in agriculture, which was the main economic activity. However, not all people wrote. The Inca of Peru, for example, had a specialized team of memory experts that kept track of communal matters of importance. You are most likely thinking about how great it would be to have such a memory. If it is any consolation, the environment we currently live in does not promote a sharp mind. Technology, stress, consumption of drugs and alcohol, poor sleep quality, and endless distractions prevent our memory from being astute.

Thereafter, in a bid to gain a peculiar identity and for ornamental purpose, people embraced art. Sculptors, painters, poets, and musicians sought to tell stories of their communities, immortalize leaders, and entertain. Architects designed unique buildings for different purposes. Therefore, agriculture not only led to civilization but has, over the years, actively supported its pillars. Despite the evolution of farming methods and technological advancement, food remains the most important aspect of human life, sustaining humanity in its entirety.

FOOD AND WAR

The beauty of the stomach is its resilience. No matter the season or the situation, it does not give up or tire. Because of this resilience, food has been an integral part of both war and civilization. We are currently living in times of attention to nutrients, counting calories, and worrying about cancer-causing substances in the food. Consider this a luxury and enjoy it while you can. You are probably thinking I should be encouraging you to eat healthily and mind calories. I will if you stick with me. Besides, I hope you will have realized how fortunate you are by then and take decisive action to eat better.

After the beginning of civilization, people were living in cities, producing adequate food, practicing religion, and creating formal governments. They were even sophisticated enough to have social classes and could write and keep records. You would think they would be content and enjoy the growing economies and prevailing peace. No, we humans are always looking for another challenge - that is how we keep developing. As expected, conflicts occurred as a result of people living together and wanting more. In some instances, the conflicts escalated into wars that got more fierce with the continual invention of sophisticated weapons.

Allow me to tell you a story. A long time ago, the world was at war. I understand there is always a war going on somewhere in the world. What I mean is a great world war. In fact, two wars. Not at the same time. The First World War started after Archduke Franz Ferdinand was assassinated in 1914 and continued until 1918, causing unprecedented levels of destruction and carnage. You would think that after losing over 16 million people to the war, humans would learn. No, your great-grandparents sat still for about 20 years, feeling dissatisfied with some unresolved issues from the first war, and decided to embark on another war that lasted from 1939 to 1945. The lives lost in World War One were not even half of those lost in the second war. Approximately 50,000,000 deaths occurred. Just so you know, these were not the only wars. There have been over 130 documented wars in history. War is the existence of a conflict between or within nations that is carried on by force of arms. Active military operations and armed conflicts mark the war period. There are, therefore, many undocumented wars in the world. The First and Second World Wars stand out merely because of the many nations involved.

HOW DOES FOOD RELATE TO WAR?

Imagine having to tend to crops while bullets are flying all around you. I doubt that you would be more concerned about your plants than your safety. However, the stomach does not understand the conflict around and will still need food. Many wars have been won and lost with food rather than guns. Militants realize that access to adequate food for both the army and the people is a prerequisite to winning a war.

During the First World War, men and horses went to the

battle, leaving farm work to the women and children. Please note that today's woman is capable of taking care of the farm. Currently, over 40 percent of the agricultural labor force in the developing world is women. However, in the old days, the division of labor was by gender. Men undertook the tough farm work like tilling the land and animal care. Women, on the other hand, took care of the children, cooked, cleaned, and sewed. If they participated in farm work, it was to sow seeds and break up clods of dirt. They were mostly not allowed to engage in economic activities, and thus, the men provided the bulk of the household needs. When the war started, the men left home, leaving women to tend to the farms and the family. They also took with them the horses that helped on the farm. As a consequence, there was a shortage of labor and, ultimately, food.

With war came transportation challenges that affected the importation of fertilizers. As a result, it became nearly impossible to access agricultural outputs. The few people who had access to the outputs began hoarding, thus driving up the prices. Therefore, even those who had adequate labor from their children did not produce optimally. Hunger lurked everywhere, stalking the civilians of the combatant countries. Consequently, some countries suffered more than others, forcing governments to take action. The result was food rationing. In Europe, the disruption of food distribution obligated the governments to oversee the delivery and the rationing to prevent the people from starvation. Long queues for food rations were a familiar scene across most of the cities in Europe.

Not everyone was fortunate enough to receive food rations. In some nations, like Turkey and Russia, there was a breakdown of the food distribution systems, leading to the starvation of many people. Similarly, Austria-Hungary lost a good number of people to hunger. The Russians did not take the dismal situation lightly. So atrocious was it that it caused the Russian Revolution.

The withholding of food by preventing its growth, post-harvest destruction, obstructing transportation, or contamination is a war tactic that has been used by different parties in history. In ancient times, armies destroyed irrigation systems and salted the ground to prevent their opposers from growing any crops. The Roman army, for example, while battling with Carthage during the Punic war, defeated the army of Hannibal, went ahead to destroy the empire, and made the land infertile by plowing it with salt. Similarly, during the American Civil War, confederate militaries dumped dead animals into the Union forces' water supplies.

Food is an essential part of human life. Without it, humans grow weak and are unable to undertake any other economic and social activities. The majority of the people today wake up early in the morning to work so they can have food on the table. Therefore, it is understandable that diet plays a significant role not only in war but also in civilization. Moreover, history has proven that food, particularly the staples, helps create and maintain large empires and strong armies.

GREAT CONQUERORS' USE OF FOODS

Food conquers the world. As absurd as it sounds, it is true. The greatest conquerors in history understood the role of food in creating and expanding their empires. They either ensured that there was adequate production or imported food from their neighbors. If you have read *The Art of War*, you know that the battle is won long before the first sword is drawn. In the same manner, these conquerors planned their attack well. Along with having well-trained armies, they recognized the power of a well-fed population and military.

Adequate food supplies were crucial in conquering other lands and people. However, its absence in the enemy's camp was terrific. Military commanders could capitalize on this shortcoming to win a battle without any fight. One such conqueror is Egypt's Thutmose III, the first to acquire the title of Pharaoh. During the Battle of Megiddo, when he fought against the King of Kadesh, Thutmose III employed the element of surprise to gain access to the fortress of Megiddo. He then built a moat and surrounded the city with wooden palisades. The occupants, starved of water and food, had to run out and surrender. Instead of taking treasures of gold and silver, the Egyptians gathered sheep, mares, cattle, foals, stallions, and prisoners that they used for labor. Food was on their mind even in victory.

A good example of a conqueror with a sound understanding of the role of food is Alexander the Great or Alexander III of Macedon. He only served as king between 336 BC and 323 BC, but he left a mark in history as the most triumphant military commander. Having ascended to power at the young age of twenty, he went on to create one of the largest ancient empires undefeated. His territory stretched from Greece to Northwest India. Being victorious in all his battles took careful planning, including adequate food supplies. The Macedonians consumed carbohydrates like millet, wheat, and barley. The grains were ground and made either into porridge or bread. Alexander exploited their ease of production, long shelf life, and nutritional value to keep his army energized. The soldiers complemented the carbohydrates with dried meat, fresh meat or shellfish when possible, and fruits. So attentive was he to the food needs of his troops that, in addition to scouting the terrain and climate, he gave exceptional focus to food availability. He knew that a good supply of food directly boosted the men's morale and efficiency on the battlefield.

Unlike Alexander the Great, whose army had to process and prepare the grains, Atilla the Hun had it easy. He was the leader of the Huns, an ancient nomadic people, and head of the Hunnic Empire. Atilla was known for his strong personality that held together his empire. Moreover, he was an astounding militant and brilliant horseman. During his reign, which lasted from 434 AD to 453 AD, he gained the reputation of a fearsome barbaric leader. The Huns were pastoral warriors and mainly ate milk and meat. They also ate tubers that they dug up as they went. There was no need for food preparation. In fact, they did not use fire at all. The only semblance of cooking was putting meat between their thighs. The vast wildlands available those days ensured that the Huns had adequate food and could keep fighting. For them, it was as simple as digging up tubers and marching forward. Ironically, there are claims that Atilla died from eating and drinking too much on his wedding day. Please learn from Atilla the Hun: do not overindulge. You could end up dead.

FOOD FOR THE MARCHING ARMIES

Carbohydrates have been fuelling armies for decades. For the Roman armies, they were the most essential source of calories. The most common staple foods were wheat and barley, which were complemented with meat. Soldiers had to hunt all available game to get adequate meat rations. Carbohydrates thus came to the rescue, providing the necessary nutrients and energy.

I do not want you to think that staple foods were only history-defining in ancient times. During the First World War, the United States believed that food would help win the war by feeding its over four million servicemen. The United States Food Administration ran campaigns to convince Americans to change their way of eating so as to feed their army in Europe. Slogans such as "Go wheatless," "Save the sugar," and "Meatless Mondays" were common. Wheat was in particularly high demand due to its high energy as well as ease of transportation. Americans were urged to eat potatoes, which were too heavy to ship. Corn was promoted as the main alternative to wheat, as it could make bread, cakes, griddle cakes, and other baked goods.

Americans were not the only ones with food on the brain. Australian authorities noted that their supreme function was to keep undisturbed the food supply from the country. Being a major supplier of both wheat and meat to Great Britain, and having the dominion troops as part of the British armed forces,

Australians had a duty to fulfill. As nature would have it, a drought occurred, causing a shortage of both wheat and meat available for export. To show the importance of providing food for the army, Australia banned their export to anywhere except Britain. The emphasis on the war effort was so great that processed wheat and meat were packed ready for shipping, crowding storage and limiting further production for the local market. By 1917, the shortage had resulted in communal uprising and industrial discontent.

For most governments, feeding the armed forces was the main priority, as they wanted to win the war. Cereals such as wheat and barley remained the staple foods for almost all armies as they were not only filling, but also nutritious. Besides, once dry, they could last for a long time and were widely produced and therefore cheap. Their versatility also helped to awaken the taste buds and break the monotony of the same bland meal. Flours could make cakes, bread, and porridge, among other things.

STAPLE FOODS IN THE CIVILIZED WORLD

The more things change, the more they remain the same. Interestingly, the staple foods that supported the early civilizations continue to support the modern world. As discussed, ancient civilizations emerged from the fruitful domestication of plants and animals. Grains such as wheat, corn, barley, millet, and peas were the main crops at the time. They were also used by the great conquerors and fed armies during war. Their role and significance in supporting a healthy life cannot be overstated. Despite all that, staple foods in the civilized world are not accorded the value they deserve.

Civilization is characterized as having cities, religion, government, social structure, writing, and art. Sadly, historians missed the most important pillar of not only civilization but also life: food. Civilization is synonymous with progress, development, enlightenment, and advancement. None of those things is associated with hungry people. Early religious leaders even offered food to the people before preaching to them. They understood that enlightenment is not possible for the hungry. In the same manner, there cannot be civilization without food. Historians should have had food production or access as the first pillar of development.

Time-proven carbohydrates are still the fuel that is in use today. Surprisingly, despite the bad reputation accorded to them, millions of people consume them each day. In the United Kingdom, the daily sale of bread is about 12 million loaves. The situation is similar in the United States, where 99.8 percent of the entire population, approximately 325 million people, eats bread. The only difference between the early days and now is the variety of products made from the grains. For example, pizza, pies, bread, pasta, burgers, cakes, cookies, breakfast cereals, soups, chips, crisps, and even salads use a form of cereal. If you have a close relationship with the bottle, you have not been left out. Vodka, gin, beer, and whiskey make use of staple foods such as wheat, potatoes, barley, corn, and rye. You now understand why life would lose flavor if we did away with good old carbohydrates.

CHAPTER SUMMARY

In summary, staple foods around the world are carbohydrates, with rice, wheat, and corn being the most popular. They have provided energy for humanity from the days of hunting and gathering, through ancient civilization and wars to modern civilization. Indeed, food has conquered nations and won wars. Today, carbohydrates continue to be the most consumed foods.

In the next chapter, you will learn more about these wonder foods. We will look at each of them in detail, paying attention to what makes them widely accepted, their nutritional value, and their calorie content.

CHAPTER FOUR: CEREALS, ROOTS, AND TUBERS

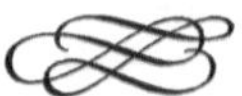

We take pride in how far humanity has come from the ancient days. We even go ahead and refer to our ancestors as being primitive. True, we are sophisticated. We have built technology to ease work and make our lives simple. We are the best form of humanity that has ever existed. Yet with all that advancement, our basic instincts are the same as our forefathers. We understand the need for each other, have conflicts, protect our families, and eat the same foods.

As we previously learned, our ancient relatives ate mainly cereals, roots, and tubers. Cereals are grasses grown for their edible seed or grain components, that is, their germ, bran, and endosperm. Examples include wheat, rice, oats, corn, rye, sorghum, and millet. Starchy roots and tubers are those plants that store nutrients, moisture, and edible starch material in tubers, roots, corms, and rhizomes. Specifically, "roots" refers to the parts of plants that grow downwards to absorb nutrients and moisture while anchoring the plant. Some of these root crops include sweet potatoes and cassava. On the other hand, tubers are enlarged underground nutrient-storing structures and include arrowroots, yams, taro, and cocoyams. Cereal grains are the main sources of carbohydrates, followed closely by root and tuber crops.

At the time of plant domestication, it made sense to bring in the same crops that humans had been feeding on for years. Similarly, despite our high level of civilization, we have not reinvented the wheel, only used it differently. Roots, tubers, and cereal grains remain the most consumed staple foods in the world. However, the specific grains and tubers vary across regions as per availability, culture, and taste preferences. To show the popularity of carbohydrates, consider that out of the over 50,000 edible plants available in the world, we get most of our energy from about 15 of them. Only this small fraction of crops provide around 90 percent of our food needs. Some examples are sorghum, millet, potatoes, yams, and cassava. That is not all. Only three crops—corn, rice, and wheat—provide for two-thirds of the world's needs. When you think about it, we are not that different from each other if you look at what we like to eat, and food does not lie.

While a majority of the people have maintained the same staple foods as their great-grandparents, others have welcomed change. Most of the time, the change is a result of changes in climate that limit the production of certain foods, advancement in agricultural technologies, better storage, and improved transportation systems. Let us face it: staples have also changed due to globalization and peer influence. How many times have you heard someone comment that they no longer consume wheat while their entire lineage lived on it? The internet has made the world accessible and bombarded us with both information and misinformation.

Our inherent obsession with carbohydrates stems from a good understanding of both the environment and our bodies. Cereal grains, tubers, and some legumes are not only packed with calories necessary for sustaining our energy needs but also full of macronutrients such as proteins, carbohydrates, and fiber.

They also contain vital minerals and vitamins like zinc, iron, calcium, and folic acid. Some of these nutrients exist in small quantities, hence the need to add other foods, such as vegetables and protein-rich foods, to your diet. There are existing negative perceptions on many of the staple foods. You may or may not have joined the bandwagon. However, before you castigate carbohydrates, let us look at what makes them popular and their nutritional value. After all, information is power.

CEREALS, ROOTS, AND TUBERS ABOVE OTHERS

The sustained use of these staple foods over the years must be for a reason. We cannot all be so crazy as to follow such a diet blindly. Well, some are. However, with increased technology and research abilities, we are in a better position to understand the continued appearance of these carbohydrates on our plates. Besides, why carbohydrates and not any other food? Let's explore the main reason we eat. Some will say, so as not to feel hungry. The truth is, hunger is annoying. However, we all need energy for body functions and to engage in physical and mental activities. Carbohydrates are sources of dietary energy, with cereals containing the most. People who engage in physical activities prefer more of these foods, which replenish the energy spent.

You eat what you sow. Cereals, for instance, can grow in various soil types and climatic conditions, and hence, feed more people. Take wheat, for example: it successfully grows in altitudes ranging from sea level to around 10,000 feet. The minimum annual amount of rainfall required for its growth is only 10 inches, which is available in most parts of the world. Relatively fertile soil is suitable for its production. Other cereals, like rye and barley, can grow in less fertile soils. Output can be improved by ensuring good humus content or adding chemical fertilizers if need be. Moreover, the harvested seeds can be replanted, making them easy to grow even in areas where farmers cannot afford or access certified seeds. Like our forefathers, modern farmers make certain the seed is free from impurities, and they are of good quality. In cases where a farmer needs to purchase cereal grains, they are easily available at an affordable cost. Most small-scale farmers plant grains meant for consumption. Additionally, many of the cereal grains grow in both spring and winter, meaning that food production is not limited by seasons. Barley and wheat are good examples.

Roots and tubers are also fairly easy to grow. You can get multiple plants from one plant. For instance, one potato plant yields about ten potatoes on average, which can be planted, thus continually increasing the area under the crop. Other crops, like cassava, are propagated cuttings. One plant can, therefore, be used to grow many others. Moreover, most root and tuber crops do well in poor soils with little water. In dry areas, roots and tubers meet the bulk of the population's energy needs. They also tend to be disease and pest-resistant, greatly reducing their cost of production. In most cases, the yield is good even under minimal management.

Since most of the staple foods produce bumper harvests, their ability to store well is crucial. Cereal grains, in particular, have a long shelf life even without processing. In reality, processing reduces their shelf life. Once they are harvested, all that is important is proper drying to reduce the moisture content that spoils them. They can either be stored as they are, as traditionally done, in a well-aerated place, or treated with pesticides to prevent pest infestation. In addition to chemical pesticides, farmers can use locally available plants with pesticidal or antimicrobial properties, like neem, mint, walnut, and turmeric. Some roots and tubers can be left underground until needed. In other areas, they are harvested, then stored in underground pits which are covered with soils and thatch. The ability of staple foods to store well for extended periods not only ensures their continued availability but also serves to cushion people in case of crop failure. The long shelf life also makes them economically viable, and hence available, in many parts of the world.

The world is a global village with all manner of foods available in different parts. Staple foods, like rice and wheat, are imported by nations that do not have adequate production. Transportation is eased by their relatively small grain sizes that are not bulky and their ability to last long. As earlier noted, wheat was one of the main crops exported during the war to feed troops and civilians in war-torn areas. Wheat, rice, and corn continue to be transported to areas with inadequate supplies, thus increasing their popularity.

As staple foods move around the globe, humans take the opportunity to experiment with them. Today, none of them has a sole use or is prepared by only one method. Since they are readily available and affordable, humans have not shied away from making them in different ways according to their culture and taste preferences. Furthermore, the increased ease of processing has contributed to even more products being made from them. Unlike in the ancient days, when making flour meant hours spent working the stone, some modern people do not even know that flour comes from grain. The processing industry has made our lives so simple that buying flour is more common than buying actual grains or tubers. If you were to give someone a choice between getting a free sack of corn grains or buying a packet of cornmeal, most people would opt to buy the flour. We prefer the easy way out. The beauty of this, however, is that these staple foods are now made into different products that appeal to our taste buds, so we keep up the consumption.

Moving away from ourselves, the popularity of cereals is also due to their being food for farm animals. Some farmers plant cereals purely for animal feed, but in many parts of the world, the plant remains keep animals full. In times when every coin counts, having an integrated farm system is beneficial. The animals eat the plant remains and give manure to apply to the crops. Such a mutually favorable system reduces the expense of buying fertilizers and planting grass for animals.

NUTRITIONAL VALUE OF CEREAL GRAINS

Grains are not merely filling foods that supply us with a high amount of energy. They consist of the endosperm, aleuronic layer, embryo, and testa. The different parts contain different nutrients. The living part of the seed is the embryo and is mainly rich in nutrients. The aleuronic layer is concentrated with vitamins, minerals, and proteins, while starch is found in the endosperm. Grains typically are sources of carbohydrates, energy, proteins, minerals, and fiber.

Most people consider grains to be pure carbohydrates with no vitamins. While they are not abundantly equipped with vitamins, they do contain vitamin E and some B vitamins like riboflavin, niacin, thiamin, and folate. In addition to vitamins, grains also contain dietary fiber that helps in the reduction of cholesterol levels in the blood. Fiber also lessens the risk of obesity, type 2 diabetes, and heart diseases. If you are one of those people who do not look forward to bowel movements, eat some grains. The fiber reduces diverticulosis and constipation, allowing you to go smoothly.

Cereals contain about 7-12 percent protein, according to the FAO. They contain different amino acids that form all kinds of proteins. Proline, glycine, and glutamine are the main amino acids that form cereal proteins such as globulins, prolamins, albumins, and glutelins. Cereal proteins are important in the formation of polymer networks during baking. Gluten gives them elasticity. Thus, these proteins are crucial in the ability of cereals to be made into different products. Below is a summary of the different amino acids found in some of the common grains.

Table 1. Amino acid composition of cereal grains; representative values in grams per 100 g protein

Amino acid	Maize	Rice	Wheat	Barley	Oats	Rye
Indispensable						
Histidine	2.6	2.4	2.3	2.1	2.1	2.2
Isoleucine	3.6	3.8	3.5	3.5	3.8	3.5
Leucine	11.1	8.2	6.7	6.7	7.2	6.2
Lysine	2.3	3.7	2.7	2.6	3.7	3.4
Methionine	1.6	2.1	1.2	1.6	1.8	1.4
Cysteine	2.0	1.6	2.5	2.2	2.7	1.9
Phenylalanine	4.4	4.8	4.6	5.1	5.0	4.5
Tyrosine	3.5	4.0	1.7	3.0	3.4	1.9
Threonine	3.3	3.4	2.8	3.4	3.4	3.4
Tryptophan	0.7	1.3	1.5	1.6	1.3	1.1
Valine	4.0	5.8	4.3	5.0	5.1	4.8

Amino acid	Maize	Rice	Wheat	Barley	Oats	Rye
Alanine	8.2	5.8	3.5	4.2	4.5	4.3
Arginine	4.4	7.5	4.3	4.8	6.2	4.6
Aspartic acid	7.2	9.6	4.9	5.6	7.7	7.2
Glutamic acid	18.6	19.2	32.1	23.5	21.0	24.2
Glycine	3.9	4.3	4.0	3.8	4.6	4.3
Proline	8.8	4.6	10.7	10.9	5.1	9.4
Serine	4.6	4.6	4.5	4.0	4.6	3.8

Source: Encyclopedia of Human Nutrition *(Price & Welch, 2013)*

Cereal grains are synonymous with carbohydrates, which are their main components. In fact, there are five groups of carbohydrates: oligosaccharides, mono and disaccharides, cell wall storage polysaccharides, storage polysaccharides, and cell wall structural polysaccharides. On average, cereals contain about 87 grams of carbohydrates for every 100 grams. We all need energy to survive and thrive. Carbohydrates are the main sources of energy for humans, contributing approximately 45-70 percent of our total energy needs. They, therefore, play a major role in homeostasis and metabolism.

Image 1: Summary of the nutritional components of major cereal grains

Cereals	Protein (%)	Fat (%)	Crude fiber (%)	Ash (%)	Starch (%)	Total dietary fiber (%)	Total phenol (mg/100 g)
Wheat	14.4	2.3	2.9	1.9	64.0	12.1	20.5
Rice	7.5	2.4	10.2	4.7	77.2	3.7	2.51
Maize	12.1	4.6	2.3	1.8	62.3	12.8	2.91
Sorghum	11	3.2	2.7	1.8	73.8	11.8	43.1
Barley	11.5	2.2	5.6	2.9	58.5	15.4	16.4
Oats	17.1	6.4	11.3	3.2	52.8	12.5	1.2
Rye	13.4	1.8	2.1	2.0	68.3	16.1	13.2
Finger millet	7.3	1.3	3.6	3.0	59.0	19.1	102
Pearl millet	14.5	5.1	2.0	2.0	60.5	7.0	51.4
Proso millet	11	3.5	9.0	3.6	56.1	8.5	–
Foxtail millet	11.7	3.9	7.0	3.0	59.1	19.11	106
Kodo millet	8.3	1.4	9.0	3.6	72.0	37.8	368

Source: Palanisamy et al (2014), "Health benefits of finger millet."

NUTRITIONAL VALUE OF ROOTS AND TUBERS

Most staple roots and tuber crops, with the exception of potatoes and sweet potatoes, have not gained adequate recognition of their dietary role. Previously dubbed "poor man's foods" and ignored, they have proven that they are not only filling but also nutritious. However, their consumption remains higher in rural communities than in urban centers. Understandably, the urban man prefers convenience and instant foods rather than tubers that mainly do not come peeled, processed or pre-cooked. Their shelf life in a city home is limited and thus a deterrent.

Roots and tubers are packed with high amounts of carbohydrates that are second only to those of cereal crops, and hence are important in keeping the world bursting with energy. In addition to this, they contain some essential vitamins and minerals, although they lose some when processed. Remember the Huns, led by Atilla the Hun? They understood this and ate them raw. In dry areas, roots and tuber crops are a major source of water helping to not only provide food but also keep the people from dehydration. A definite benefit of the roots and tubers is their ability to multitask. For many of them, the leaves are edible and contribute to added nutritional value. For example, cocoyam, sweet potato, and cassava leaves are rich in vitamins, minerals, and proteins.

Table 2: Nutritional components of common roots and tubers					
Nutrients (per 100 g)	Potatoes		Sweet potatoes, raw	Cassava, raw	Yam, raw
	White flesh and skin, raw	Red flesh and skin, raw			
Proximate composition					
Energy (kcal)	69.0	70	86.0	160.0	118.0
Protein (g)	1.7	1.9	1.6	1.4	1.5
Total lipid (fat) (g)	0.1	0.1	0.1	0.3	0.2
Carbohydrate, by difference (g)	15.7	15.9	20.1	38.1	27.9
Fiber, total dietary (g)	2.4	1.7	3.0	1.8	4.1
Sugars, total (g)g	1.2	1.3	4.2	1.7	0.5

Nutrients (per 100 g)	Potatoes		Sweet potatoes, raw	Cassava, raw	Yam, raw
	White flesh and skin, raw	Red flesh and skin, raw			
Minerals					
Calcium, Ca (mg)	9	10	30	16	17
Magnesium, Mg (mg)	21	22	25	21	21
Potassium, K (mg)	407	455	337	271	816
Phosphorus, P (mg)	62	61	47	27	55
Sodium, Na (mg)m	16	18	55	14	9

Nutrients (per 100 g)	Potatoes		Sweet potatoes, raw	Cassava, raw	Yam, raw
	White flesh and skin, raw	Red flesh and skin, raw			
Vitamins					
Total ascorbic acid (mg)	19.70	8.60	2.40	20.60	17.10
Thiamin (mg)	0.07	0.08	0.08	0.09	0.11
Riboflavin (mg)	0.03	0.03	0.06	0.05	0.03
Niacin (mg)	1.07	1.15	0.56	0.85	0.55
Vitamin B-6 (mg)	0.203	0.170	0.209	0.088	0.293
Folate (μg-DFE)	18	18	11	27	23
Vitamin E (mg)	0.01	0.01	0.26	0.19	0.35
Vitamin K (μg)	1.6	2.9	1.8	1.9	2.3
Vitamin A (IU)IU	8	7	14187	13	138

Source: USDA

CHAPTER SUMMARY

You now know that staple foods are not only rich in carbohy-drates meant to energize us but also contain vitamins, proteins, fiber, and various minerals. They do more than keep us satisfied. Besides, staple foods are not mean - they aim to serve as many people as possible by growing in a wide range of altitudes and weather conditions. Roots and tubers take this further by doing well even in areas with poor soils and little rainfall. Moreover, staple foods have long shelf lives and are most convenient to transport.

In the next chapter, you will learn about how humans have altered staple foods to appeal to their taste preferences and love for ease and convenience. Yes, we love delicious food and are willing to experiment. Not all of us - some prefer as little work as possible.

CHAPTER FIVE: POTATOES, PASTA, COOKED RICE AND BREAD

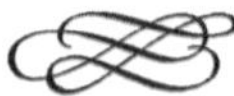

ood is not only a necessity, but also a pleasure to enjoy. The appreciation for food is not solely dependent on its kind, but also on how it is prepared. In some cultures, eating is an experience and part of the social setting. Over the years, staple foods have been altered into different forms to meet our dietary and palatability needs. Before the discovery of fire, meals were taken raw, but that is no longer the case. Let us explore the different ways of preparing staple foods and how they have changed over the years.

ALTERATION OF FOODS

Initially, most foods were eaten in their natural state as much as possible. Our ancestors may have had such deep respect for food that they opted not to alter it, or they lacked the know-how. To date, there are still some staple foods consumed with minimal alterations. Cassava, yams, and sweet potatoes are some examples. Our ancestors invented cooking about 2 million years ago. The earliest hearths are estimated to be at least 790,000 years old. Archaeological evidence dating back to approximately

300,000 years ago indicates the presence of earth ovens, ancient fireplaces, flint, and burnt animal bones.

After the discovery of fire, it was only natural that the oldest method of cooking was open-fire roasting. While many of us enjoy grilled foods using modern equipment, in those days food was placed directly into the fire, ashes, and all. Some communities still use this method of cooking. There is a possibility that despite the medicinal value of ashes, some people did not enjoy them as food accompaniments, hence the shift to suspending food over a fire. Others used fire pits for cooking.

The Aurignacian people from southern France steamed food by wrapping it in wet leaves and placing it over hot embers. From there, humans engaged in toasting wild grains by placing them on flat rocks, and heating liquids in shells, hollow stones, and skulls. In the absence of pots, anything cooked. The introduction of earthenware, the domestication of plants and animals, and a dependable food supply broadened culinary techniques. Wheat and barley were the first to be processed by grinding them on a stone before baking them into seed cakes. Grinding and baking were essential developments for humanity's nutrition, as they aided the uptake of carbohydrates into the blood. Currently, in addition to roasting, baking, and steaming, other methods used in food preparation are boiling, pickling, frying, baking, stewing, dry and wet milling, flaking, fermentation, sprouting, brewing, extrusion, and braising. Other people opt for poaching, simmering, grilling, broiling, and blanching.

The industrial processing of foods, especially cereals, into flour and other products has dramatically contributed to the increased ways of food preparation. Except for roots and tubers that make their way to the kitchen in their natural state, most foods are processed and packed. The processing of grains allows for different styles of cooking. For example, wheat is made into all-purpose flour, bread flour, cake flour, and self-rising flour. All these are used for different purposes. Additionally, there is the fortification of food, the addition of flavor, and the removal of undesired contents.

MAKING COMPOUND DISHES

As humanity advanced, the first compound dish was made: a coarse paste of cracked kernels of wild grasses mixed with water before being toasted on a stone and voilà, the first bread! Like most things historical, we can't say much about it with certainty. However, our forefathers did combine different ingredients to create exciting foods. Ashishim, a red lentil pancake, is among the earliest recorded compound dishes from ancient Israel. Other old dishes include bread (focaccia, flatbread, and mantou), hardtack, harissa, oatcake, and noodles. While there have been few modifications from the original recipes, many of the dishes are still made. Some other significant compound dishes include bread, pasta, tortillas, fufu, and naan.

Bread is the most commonly consumed food in the world, providing a significant source of carbohydrates. A contributing factor in its popularity is the ability to be made using flour from different grains such as wheat, rye, rice, oats, corn, millet, flax, and spelt. We have come a long way from the first bread, which was mainly gruel cooked on a stone, to soft, sweet, and fluffy bread. The basic modern process of making bread is similar to the ancient one and involves mixing flour, water, and yeast, or none into a dough then baking. Leavening and the use of refined flours allow the bread to rise and be soft. Nevertheless, unleavened bread called flatbreads is still a favorite in some regions. There are variations to the basic recipe, like adding butter, milk, salt, or sugars, depending on one's preference. The mechanized slicing of bread introduced by Otto Rohwedder in 1928 has also been a welcomed invention.

Bread was not the only dish made by mixing flour with other ingredients. Corn tortillas, an ancient intervention, are estimated to have been first prepared around 10,000 BC. The time coincides with the early domestication of corn. The tortilla is a thin flatbread made from finely ground corn and water then cooked on a griddle. Closely related to tortillas is naan from Asia, a kind of bread made from combining wheat, water, yeast, and sugar and cooked on a skillet with or without oil or butter.

Roots and tubers have not been left behind. Africans invented fufu, a traditional meal that is made by boiling yams, cassava, plantains, or a mixture of these, then pounding them until they are smooth. A variation of fufu similarly uses corn-meal flour to yield pap or ugali. The combination of ingredients also works with meat. Pemmican, for example, is made by pounding dried meat into a powder then mixing it with melted fat. In some instances, dried berries such as blueberries, currants, and cherries are added. Pemmican is an ideal source of energy and proteins.

USE OF SPICES AND HERBS

Having a steady supply of food was only the first step to improving our cuisine. Over the years, humans have used roots, fruits, seeds, barks, leaves, flowers, and other plant substances to flavour or garnish food. Egyptians, Indians, and the Chinese were the first people to use spices and herbs. Some of the earliest used spices are cinnamon and black pepper in the Middle East and herbs and pepper in East Asia. By 1700 BC, cloves were also commonly used in Mesopotamia. Today, there are over 100 different spices, with nutmeg, ginger, pepper, cinnamon, turmeric, garlic, paprika, chili, oregano, and cumin being some of the most popular. Herbs and spices not only impart flavor, but also add zest to food and stimulate the appetite. Besides, they have some health benefits. Garlic, for example, lowers blood pressure, while cayenne pepper helps in burning fat.

BREAD, LOAVES, AND FLATBREADS

As early as 800 BC, Egyptians were making bread by crushing grain using a quern. Today, bread is a staple food in many homes and eaten by every culture, race, and religion. For instance, every American consumes about 53 pounds of bread annually. In the West and Greater Middle East, bread is a staple food with cultural significance that goes beyond nutritive value. In medieval times, England had a law stipulating hefty punishments for short-changing bakers. So politically significant is bread that inflation in its price in the nineteenth century caused major divisions in Britain. The United Kingdom consumes about 12 million loaves a day. The versatility of bread contributes to its elevated status on the plate. There are different types of bread for different regions and purposes.

In Asia, the Chinese have traditional mantou, an alternative staple to rice in northern and central China. Indians have chapati, naan, and roti, while the Philippines have pandesa, also called salt bread. The popularity and variety of bread in Europe is staggering. Germans alone have more than 300 types, with each person estimated to eat an average of 53 kilograms annually. Conversely, baguette culture in France is on the decline. The average consumption of bread is only half a loaf per day, as compared to about three loaves a century ago. In Latin America, flatbreads are typical, with sopaipillas being the most popular. The region's top bread consumer is Chile, which also takes the second position worldwide. Ethiopians and Egyptians are also heavy bread consumers.

PASTA AND NOODLES

The similarity between pasta and noodles opens up the debate on who is the copycat. Have you ever wondered which came first, Italian pasta or Chinese noodles? There is no conclusive evidence. A common belief is that it was Marco Polo who introduced pasta to Italians after exploring the Far East in the thirteenth century. However, archaeological evidence from an Etruscan tomb dated to 4000 BC shows a possible indication of pasta, while Chinese noodles are thought to be from around 3000 BC. The debate goes on.

Originally, pasta was made with durum wheat flour, also called semolina, mixed with water. In other times, farina, coarse granulations of various high-quality hard wheat, was used. Today, some people use wheat flour in pasta making. Coloring uses vegetable juices, tomatoes, beef, or tomato mixture where necessary. The addition of herbs and spices boosts flavor. The dough is rolled and pasteurized before cutting into the desired shape and sizes. Noodles, on the other hand, use ordinary wheat flour, and the dough goes through sheeting where it is made into a flat sheet before cutting. The main difference is texture and taste. Pasta's texture is "al dente," firm at the core but soft on the outside.

Both pasta and noodles have gained worldwide acceptance and are consumed in many parts of the world. South Korea tops the list of noodle-consuming nations at about 75 servings per person per year, followed by Vietnam at 54 servings and Nepal at 53 servings. China alone accounts for 39 percent of global consumption. In general, there are around 290 million servings of noodles eaten each day. Unlike the Chinese, the Italians love pasta, consuming about 23.5 kilograms per capita. Other pasta lovers are Tunisia at 17 kilograms, Venezuela at 12 kilograms, and Greece at 11 kilograms. Americans consume 24 percent of the world's pasta, about 6 billion pounds per year.

RICE

The Chinese are believed to be the first to domesticate rice around the upper Huai and middle Yangtze valleys about 8,000 years ago. Other early cultivators of rice are Indians and Sri Lankans, before it spread to the rest of the world. Today, production stands at roughly 499 million metric tonnes and its popularity on the rise. The global consumption stands at approximately 486.62 million metric tonnes up from 437 million metric tonnes recorded in 2009. The top rice-consuming nation is China, with 143 million metric tonnes, followed by India with 100 million metric tonnes. Rice is the second most grain produced in the world, after corn.

While there are many ways of preparing rice, a basic method is to boil it and eat it with other accompanying dishes. Conversely, some familiar stand-alone rice dishes include risotto (Italy), nasi goreng (Indonesia), jollof rice (West Africa), fried rice (China), and biryani (India). Other products, like cakes and porridge, are made using rice flour.

FUFU

Believed to have its origin in Ghana, fufu is made using a starchy food crop like yam, cassava, or plantains. Fufu means any starch that is mashed or ground and cooked into a creamy paste. Cassava fufu is popular in Sierra Leone, Côte D'Ivoire, Ghana, Togo, Nigeria, Benin, and Liberia. Some variations of fufu are kokonte, made from black yam, ugali, made from cornmeal, matoke, made from plantains, and banku, made from corn and cassava.

POTATOES AND YAMS

Potatoes have their origin in the Peruvian and Bolivian Andes. Nearly 1,800 years ago, they were primarily cultivated by the Incas in South America before their introduction into Europe in the sixteenth century. They became a significant crop in Ireland, Germany, and the west of England by the close of the eighteenth century before spreading to the rest of the world. And we embraced them in all manners: boiled, baked, stewed, fried, and made into a wide range of dishes. Popular potato products include French fries, potato chips, soups, pancakes, and dumplings.

Each person is estimated to consume around 110 pounds of potatoes each year. Despite warnings from health workers, particularly on fried potato products, the potato remains among the top four most important staple crops after wheat, maize, and rice. The global production is over 300 million metric tonnes. Interestingly, China is the highest producer, at 99 million tonnes, and consumer, at 61 million tonnes, of potatoes annually. Other countries, like India, Russia, and Ukraine, are also significant producers. Belarus boasts the highest per capita consumption of potatoes at 178 kilograms, with Ukraine and Latvia following.

The yam is native to Africa and quite popular in West Africa, where in addition to being the primary staple food, it is the focal point for cultural rituals. Nigeria produces over 70 percent of yams globally, 44 million tonnes, followed by Ghana at 7.4 million tonnes and the Ivory Coast at 5.9 million tonnes. As well as being the largest producers, Africans are the main consumers. Other countries that appreciate their nutritional value include Brazil, Colombia, Vietnam, the Philippines, Japan, India, Indonesia, and Jamaica. Yams are mainly made into fufu, but they can also be roasted, fried, or baked, similar to potatoes. The yam derives its name from a word meaning "eating," yet it is not globally eaten as much as it should be, considering its nutritional value and health benefits.

CHAPTER SUMMARY

In summary, humanity has been altering food for centuries and will continue to do so as the environment, technology, and taste preferences change.

In the next chapter, we look at modern farming, current production, global trends, and systems used.

CHAPTER SIX: FARMING PRACTICES OF TODAY

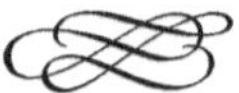

If you lived in an ancient civilization, would you be a farmer? You would have only simple tools like rakes, hoes, winnowing scoops, flint-bladed sickles, and the most sophisticated tool, the plow. If you were fortunate, your plow would be drawn by oxen. Otherwise, you would need to eat a heavy meal. Before you complain, remember that farming pioneers used sticks and hands yet produced bountiful harvests. You can relax - you live in the modern world with mechanized agriculture. Farmers have come a long way from the initial plant domestication process. Not only has the number of crops grown increased, but so have the methods of growing them.

HOW MUCH DO STAPLE FOODS ACCOUNT FOR WORLDWIDE?

Despite having 13.4 billion hectares on the planet to use in feeding ourselves, we only use 12 percent of them for crop production, 35 percent hosts woodland and grassland, and 28 percent is under forests. It's fortunate that not all land is suitable for agriculture, otherwise, animals, water bodies, and natural vegetation would need to find another planet. Only about 36 percent of the earth is, to an extent, suitable for crop production, which translates to 50 percent of the habitable land. There is, therefore, room for expansion of agriculture, although due care of the environment is paramount.

As the population multiplies, so does the demand for food. We live to eat or eat to live, depending on one's point of view. As a consequence of the growing number of humans, the area under cultivation has increased over the years. In 1961, it was 1369 million hectares, but by 2009, the figure had risen to 1527 million hectares. However, there is a small decline in areas under rain-fed agriculture but an increase in the land under irrigation. UNESCO estimates that 20 percent of cultivated land is under irrigated agriculture, which produces 40 percent of food globally. The 80 percent of agriculture that is fed by rain produces the remaining 60 percent.

Cereal grains remain the most grown crops in the world. In 1961, the total area of land producing cereal grains was 513 million hectares, but by 2017, it stood at 731 million hectares. Wheat is the most extensively grown cereal, taking up about 17 percent of the land. According to the FAO, developing countries produce over 45 percent of the world's wheat. Around 215 million hectares of land are under the crop to cater to the more than 2.5 billion people spread across 89 countries who consume wheat and wheat products. Like that of wheat, maize production is high in developing countries, which are home to 73 percent of the approximately 200 million hectares on which it is planted. Some countries in Asia and Africa generally record low yields of below three tonnes per hectare. Barley occupies about 70 million hectares globally, with 25 percent of it grown in developing countries.

Image 6.1: Land area under cereal production (ha)

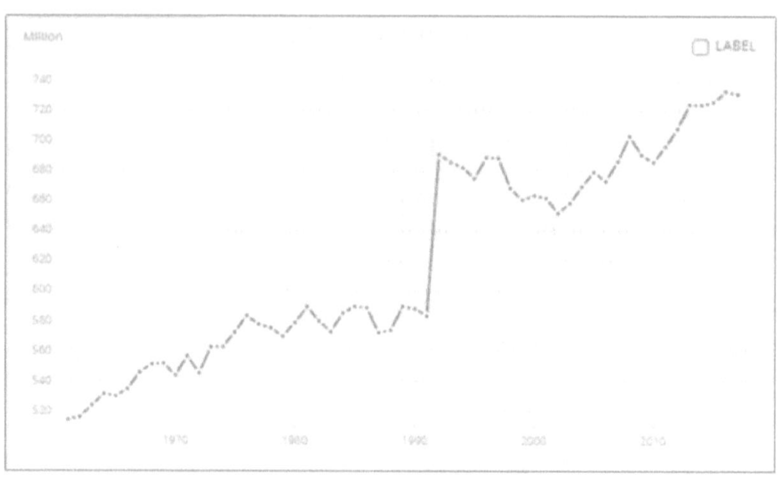

Source: The World Bank

Image 6.2: World Area harvested for various cereal grains (1961-2018)

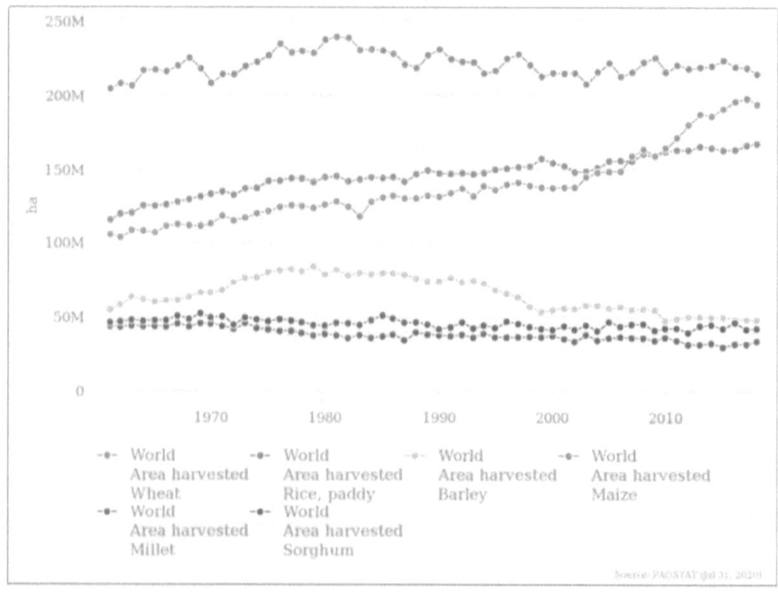

Roots and tubers have enjoyed increased acreage and production over time. People, particularly those in dry areas, are realizing their capability to produce more than cereal grains. Besides, increased research and public awareness of their satiating and nutritional value have significantly reduced their reputation as a poor man's diet. The production of roots and tubers has nearly doubled since the 1960s to reach about 800 million tonnes. The area used for these crops has seen drastic changes. Cassava farming has notably increased from less than 10 million hectares in 1961 to about 24.5 million hectares in 2018. Conversely, the area used for potato farming is on the decline, but its yield per hectare is on the rise, unlike that of other major roots and tubers. Sweet potatoes, cassava, and yams are mainly produced in developing countries. Although adapted to harsh weather, the decline in yields is attributable to climate change, low traditional knowhow on such foods, poor soils, and lack of concentration. In most cases, they are planted for subsistence use, and hence, lack of focused care. The truth is, despite the increasing acceptance of roots and tubers, most of them are still developing-world foods, eaten as an alternative to maize, rice, and wheat.

Image 6.3: World's production of roots and tubers 1961-2017

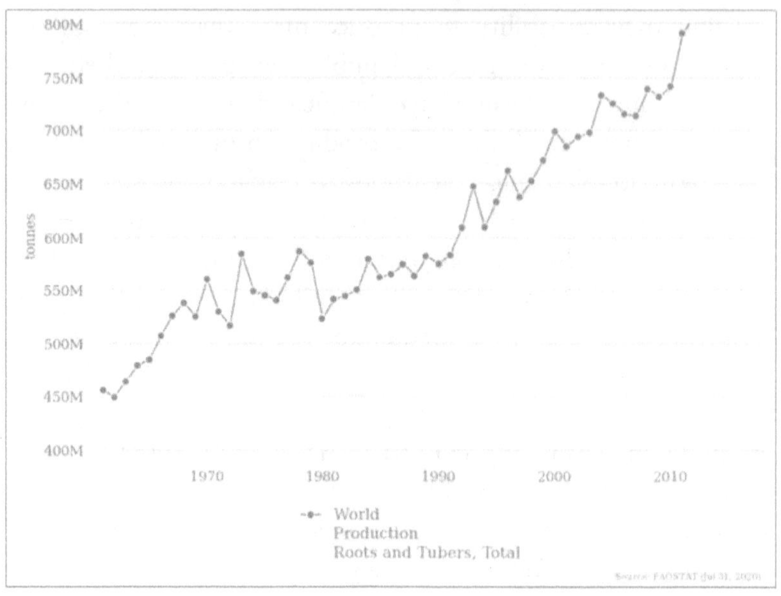

Source: FAO

Image 6.4: World area harvested for main roots and tubers

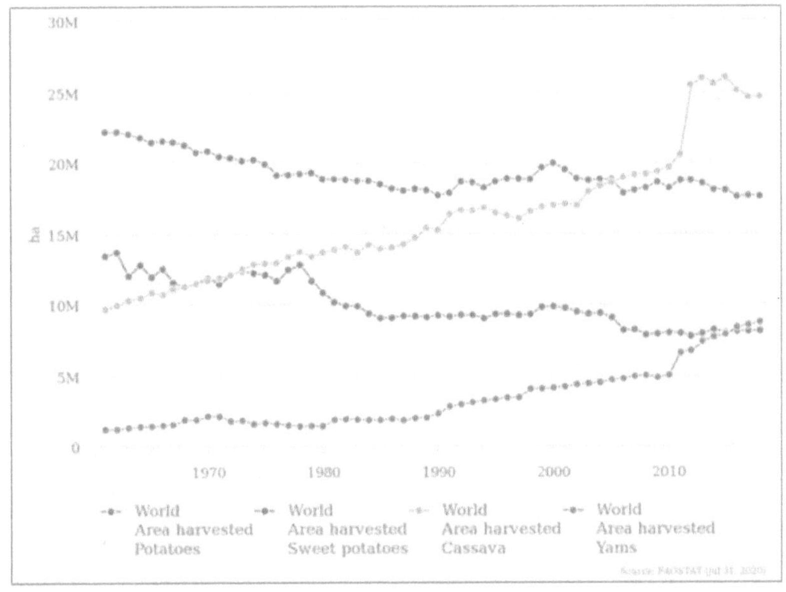

Image 6.5: Yields of roots and tubers per hectare

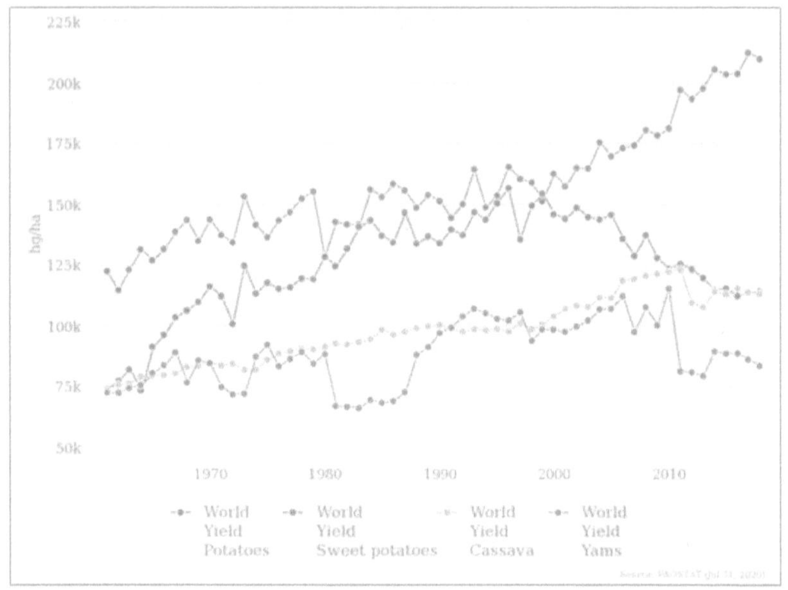

Source: FAO

ARE THEY WORTH IT?

While technological advancement has ensured that farming is more efficient than it was earlier in history, there are costs associated. Generally, the farming of staple foods under the rain-fed system is not as costly as irrigation but does not guarantee high yields. Additionally, staples grow in most soils and thus can be extensively produced. Many of these foods are widely adaptable and do well in varying temperatures. The main costs involved in the planting of cereal grains include land preparation, fertilizers, and pesticides. Roots and tubers are even better suited for growth in different climates and require minimal inputs. Thus, the overall production of these staple foods is low, particularly on a large scale.

The main staple foods, such as wheat, maize, rice, and potatoes, are bulk suppliers of carbohydrates for both humans and animals. In the United States, corn is mainly produced for animal feeds. Additionally, they are used industrially in paper production, pharmaceutical and cosmetic processes, the wood industry, textile manufacturing, and food manufacturing. They serve as adhesives, texture agents, fillers, and binders, among other uses. Therefore, they serve many other duties besides feeding the world.

Carbohydrates can be found in other foods, such as vegetables and meats. However, the amount found in vegetables is low, while meat is an expensive commodity. Additionally, the number of animals available for meat can hardly sustain the world's protein requirements and hence cannot meet our carbohydrate needs. A competitive alternative to starchy staple foods is pulse crops, which include beans, cowpeas, soybeans, peas, mung beans, and peanuts. They are also known as grain legumes. They have relatively high carbohydrate content. However, not only is their cost of production high, but their yields tend to be low. In ideal conditions, pulses yield between one-third and half of the yields of maize. They are easily affected by pest problems like angular leaf spot, bacterial blight, rust, and mosaic virus. In many farms, legumes are mainly intercropped with cereal grains to complement farmers' diets and fix nitrogen in the soil.

Table 3: Comparison of the nutritional value of cereal grains and legumes

Crop	Maize	Millet	Sorghum	Yellow beans	Raw peanuts	Cowpeas	Cassava	Potatoes (red)
Protein (g)	8.8	11	11	22	26	24	1.4	1.9
Calories/100 grams	364	378	329	345	567	343	160	70
Carbohydrates (g)	74	73	72	61	16	60	38	16

Legumes have the nutritional potential to rival cereal grains, roots, and tubers. Not only do they contain a high protein content, but they are also high in calories and carbohydrates. However, their production cannot sustainably meet the carbohydrate needs of the human population, let alone animals. You do not have to believe me. Look at the graph below. Numbers don't lie. The production of pulses is quite low and has barely increased over three decades. We love money and food. If either meat, legumes, or vegetables were a better option, we would be producing in huge quantities.

Image 6.6: Production of cereal grains, pulses, and roots and tubers in the world

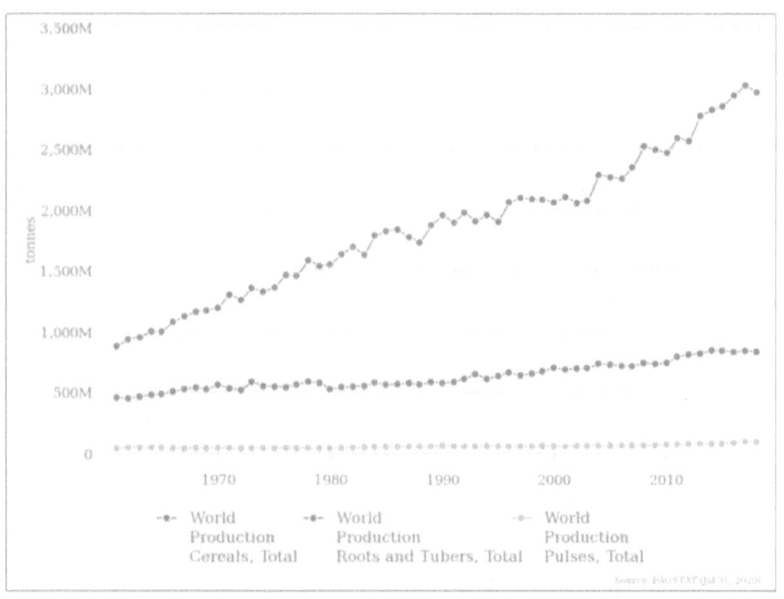

Farm Inputs: pesticides, fertilizers, and GMOs

FERTILIZERS

Farming today is synonymous with the high usage of pesticides and fertilizers. Thanks to them, food production has continually increased since the days of ancient civilizations. The quality is another issue. Most of our agricultural land has little to none of the essential nutrients necessary for optimal production of staple foods, such as potash, phosphate, and nitrogen. Fertilizers come either in liquid, solid, or gaseous forms, and contain one or more plant nutrients. Farmers have to fertilize either annually or seasonally since plants uptake them. Any excess nutrients are lost through leaching, runoff, volatilization, or emission to the air. The global application of fertilizers has been on the increase, with 107,659 kilotons of nitrogen, 47,222 kilotons of phosphate, and 37,834 kilotons of potash consumed in 2017, according to the International Fertilizer Association (IFA). By supplying the essential nutrients, fertilizers help to boost yields and thus contribute to food security and sustainable agricultural production. Today, good farm practices encourage the application of mineral fertilizers, livestock manure, crop residues, compost, and biological nitrogen fixation.

Most cereal grains require starter fertilizers, mainly nitrogen and phosphorus, for good yields. Other necessary nutrients include potassium, iron, zinc, manganese, boron, and copper. Most farmers opt to apply mineral fertilizers because they are readily available and contain specific nutrients in known quantities, unlike organic fertilizers. Roots and tubers tend to produce high yields, so they extract high levels of nutrients from the soil. Farmers should replenish these through fertilizers, but they often do not. There is an expectation that they should somehow manage to grow and give forth bountifully because they are hardy crops.

PESTICIDES

Statistics from the FAO indicate that 4,113,591 kilotons of pesticides were used in 2017. High consumption is understandable since there are many pests and diseases that affect crops. Cereal grains, in particular, face attacks from insects and worms such as aphids, thrips, grasshoppers, rice weevils, cutworms, and armyworms. Some of the major diseases include stem rust, glume blotch, leaf rust, powdery mildew, and loose smut. In the United States, corn is one of the main consumers of pesticides. Many cereal-producing countries use fungicides, herbicides, insecticides, and plant growth regulators to protect crops. Due to the damage that can arise from the use of pesticides, they are regulated and have to be approved before release to the market. Unfortunately, this does not prevent their abuse. Pesticide residue is a major issue, and adverse health effects on humans and animals are attributed to it. Environmentalists point out the soil, air, and water pollution that occur as a result of pesticide use. However, for many of us, the end justifies the means. Given a choice between the long-term effects of both fertilizers and pesticides and reduced production, we would rather eat now. We can do everything else afterward.

GENETICALLY MODIFIED ORGANISMS (GMOS)

If there is a debate that has no end in sight, it must be the GMO one. As earlier said, we love challenges and prefer to have our way. We do something about anything we do not like. For instance, someone did not like that apples browned, so he created one that did not. We are problem-solvers, but do not know where and when to stop. We now have organisms with artificially modified genetic materials that do not naturally occur. Proponents of GMOs argue that they are high-yielding, offer farmers better economics, and decrease environmental strain. On the other hand, opponents cite the threats GMOs have on biodiversity, resultant health effects such as obesity, and trade impacts.

Despite the debate, farmers are embracing GMOs. The area producing GM crops in 2014 was about 182 million hectares from 1.7 million hectares in 1996. The vast majority of GM crops are maize, soybean, canola, and cotton. Over 90 percent of corn grown in the USA today is genetically engineered. Globally, GMO maize accounts for 30 percent of the total maize grown. While most of the other staples do not have GM varieties, potatoes do. The GM potato has been in existence since 2015 and is modified to reduce bruising and to have reduced acrylamide levels when cooked. In total, GM crops occupy about 4 percent of agricultural land and are grown by less than 1 percent of farmers in the world.

DO CEREAL GRAINS AND ROOTS AND TUBERS CONTRIBUTE TO A BETTER STANDARD OF LIVING?

Poor farmers! You have probably heard that before, but never really stopped to think about it. Despite the hard work they put in, most of them do not reap profits equivalent to their sweat. In fact, if we literally ate our sweat, farmers would always be full. The global agriculture industry is worth a whopping $2.4 trillion and employs over a billion people. Yet the actual driver of the industry is barely recognized and rewarded. Not all farmers are poor, but neither are most of them rich. They receive a lot of revenue but spend much of it on inputs. Cereals, root, and tubers are not high-value crops, but they make up for that by being in steady demand and being easy to produce. The world trade in staple foods is not constant - availability determines price. In good seasons, when produce is plentiful, prices come down, and in bad years they rise. Since most staple foods have a long shelf life, farmers with the ability to store crops can cash in when prices are high.

Arguably, farmers have a good standard of living, with access to food, good health, stable mental state, low stress levels, and settled life. However, small-scale farmers are not wealthy. Production of staple foods is profitable on a large scale. As earlier discussed, farmers in parts of Asia and Africa produce less than 3 tonnes of maize per hectare, which does not give a high return on investment. Besides, the low quantities produced do not give them a competitive voice, and many rely on middlemen who offer low prices. In such areas where cereal grains have low yields, farmers should opt for roots and tubers that do well, then trade these for grains.

LOCALLY AVAILABLE RESOURCES

An advantage of staple foods is the ease of production. Farmers not only are able to use local markets to sell products, but can also purchase inputs. While there is intense marketing of certified seeds, farmers have the option of planting traditional varieties that are hardy. In most rural communities, it is normal for people to obtain seeds and planting materials from each other. Besides, farmers can use manure and compost from their farms and apply organic pesticides. Modern farming does not necessarily mean ignoring the locally available resources for expensive inputs with a certification symbol. Farmers have embraced what works for them in terms of reducing costs, improving productivity, and safeguarding human health and the environment.

CHAPTER SUMMARY

We have learned that the demand for staple foods is high. Farmers are using available technology and methods to improve production. While GMOs are slowly being embraced, the use of pesticides and fertilizer is at a global high.

In the next chapter, you will learn about what to look for while shopping for staple foods, with a focus on the most confusing food items.

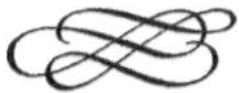

*L*et's go shopping! Not everyone likes to shop. Some face the need to shop with sheer dread. However, we need to eat food, so we have to buy it. What to pick, what not to pick, and why are some of the key questions. The shelves in stores today are packed with all kinds of products - do not be ignorant. Use your head, a bit of heart, and most importantly, your eyes to read the labels. As a bonus, you can apply my grandmother's rule: buy as natural as possible, which translates to foodstuffs with as few ingredients as possible.

TODAY'S STORE-BOUGHT BREAD VS. BREAD OF THE PAST

There is all manner of bread found in your local store, unless you live in a small town with one bakery. Even then, there is bound to be variety. Unlike bread of the past that was made with basic ingredients, stores have super-soft varieties, some flavored, forti-fied, or made with different flours. The change in store-bought bread is mainly the ingredients. Many of them have excess preservatives and emulsifiers to keep the bread soft and fresh for long. When did you last throw away a store-bought loaf of bread because it got spoiled? Stores are convenient for many of us, but extra caution is necessary while picking a loaf of bread.

MOIST VS DRY BREAD

Can you smell that? I am referring to the tantalizing aroma of a freshly baked loaf of bread. Have you tried it still warm with butter and a hot cup of tea? Moist bread's soft and fluffy texture makes it appealing to the taste buds. Dry bread, on the other hand, works well for some dishes like bread pudding, French toast, and stuffing. There are many ways of using day-old bread to get your carbon fix and enjoy it as well. When shopping, it is recommended that you choose your bread according to your need. However, if you are unable to finish a loaf of bread, don't sweat it - you can store it for later use.

WHITE VS BROWN BREAD

Did you know that traditionally, white bread was for the wealthy? Today, white bread is still a winner despite the health concerns associated with it. Brown bread uses 100 percent whole wheat and other ingredients for softness, taste, and color. As such, it is fiber-rich, but lacks that amazing aroma of ferulic acid. Conversely, white bread uses bleached flour, which gives it a distinct taste, in addition to other ingredients like color, yeast, and salt. White bread's crust also gives off chemicals that smell like caramel and potatoes, and hence are more appealing to consumers. Additionally, white bread is soft due to being more processed than brown bread. The fiber content is negligible, but brown bread contains more calories than white bread. To improve brown bread's appeal, some manufacturers add salt and sugar, which compromises its nutritional value. Generally, white bread is suitable for athletes and very active people. Your choice is between health and taste. You know what to choose, but can you do it?

WHOLE WHEAT VS WHOLE WHEAT GRAIN

The confusion that comes with shopping increases with new products each day. When shopping, do you struggle with all the differences in the items? Variety is the spice of life! However, it can be nerve-racking. In short, whole wheat is the wheat kernel that is intact, unaltered, and not mixed with other grains. Whole wheat grain, on the other hand, is wheat in its original form, including the germ, endosperm, and the nutrient-packed bran. Whole wheat grain is more nutritious and keeps us fuller because it takes longer for our bodies to digest it.

WHITE RICE VS. WILD RICE

Wild rice is not actual rice, but a type of grass that originated in America. Its naming is related to its appearance since it looks like rice. It is low in calories, high in proteins, and contains the nine essential amino acids. Moreover, it is a source of antioxidants, fiber, and nutrients such as phosphorus, magnesium, and manganese. You may need to pay more for all the benefits of wild rice. White rice is milled to remove the bran, husk, and germ to alter texture, flavor, appearance. The milling is also useful in preventing spoilage. Since we love clean, white, and polished products, the rice is also polished to give it an attractive, shiny appearance. Our forefathers would be astounded at the lengths we go to have beautiful food. They enjoyed the food in its natural state and understood that it is the soil and "dirt" that made it nutritious. Before the argument on not being our ancestors and times being different starts, it is essential to note that the polishing and milling remove nutrients. Basing your diet on un-enriched white rice exposes you to beriberi, a neurological disease caused by thiamine (Vitamin B_1) deficiency. There are laws in parts of the country that require the enrichment of white rice with some B vitamins. If you choose white rice, check on the packet to see if it is enriched.

SWEET POTATO, YAM, AND WHITE POTATO

Many roots and tubers are becoming increasingly popular. However, many of us still face confusion while shopping, particularly in differentiating between yams and sweet potatoes. Yams look like the traditional male version of sweet potatoes: rough, scaly, and difficult to peel without heat. The skin color of yams ranges from dark brown to light pink. In addition to coming in all shapes and sizes, their taste is starchy and potato-like, not quite sweet. Yams are very nutritious and contain more of several nutrients than sweet potatoes: fiber, vitamins B_6, C, and E, fats, and potassium. They will keep you full for a long time. As its name suggests, the sweet potato is sweeter than yams or potatoes. They are also attractive in either rose, red, pale copper, or purple skins with tapered ends. Sweet potatoes are also nutrient-rich, with more protein, calcium, sugar, Vitamin A, sodium, beta-carotene, and water than yams. White potatoes are all-purpose and widely consumed. They are either oblong or round in shape with a thin golden-colored skin and a waxy white or yellow flesh. They have a similar amount of carbohydrates to sweet potatoes but less fiber. Yams, white potatoes, and sweet potatoes are used in different dishes, and their flavor can be adjusted through seasoning.

TYPES OF CORN

Corn is one of the top energy-giving foods in the world. Before going shopping, you may want to know there are several types of corn, with the most common being dent corn, flint corn, popcorn, and sweet corn. These types have different uses. You don't want to be boiling popcorn.

Dent or field corn is widely grown as a livestock feed, although it is also a component of some food products. Once dry, its hard and soft starches become indented, thus its name. If you are looking for corn for decoration, then flint corn, with its hard shell and wide range of colors, will do the job. If you enjoy eating corn, then sweet corn should be on your shopping list. Also called corn on the cob, sweet corn is mainly starch and contains more sugar than all others. Unlike the other types, it is picked and consumed during the milk stage when kernels are tender, and the ears are still immature. Sweet corn does not pop like the typical popcorn. Movie lovers and parents know of the popcorn, which is also a type of flint corn without the many colors. Unlike sweet corn, popcorn has a hard outer shell but a soft starchy center. The natural moisture in the corn steams when heated, building up pressure and causing it to pop, hence the name. Popcorn is a common snack strongly associated with movies.

POPULAR GRAINS

Most people do not buy whole grains and instead opt for their processed products. However, if you are one of those people appreciative enough of good food to purchase them, then you should also prepare to shop. Oats, some of the healthiest grains, are available in many stores. They contain carbohydrates, fiber, protein, fat, vitamins, and other minerals like copper, manganese, iron, zinc, folate, and phosphorus. Another healthy option is whole-grain rye, which is more nutrient-rich than wheat with more minerals, fewer carbs, and an incredibly high amount of fiber, about 22.6 grams in a 100-gram serving. Buckwheat is also a great pick while shopping. Despite its name, it is not a relative of wheat, but a pseudocereal packed with many nutrients like copper, iron, vitamin B, fiber, and magnesium. To top that up, it is naturally gluten-free! If those do not appeal to you, there are many other options like whole barley, spelt, quinoa, millet, and cracked wheat.

CHAPTER SUMMARY

Staple foods are available in different types and forms. In most cases, it is a matter of health versus taste, and the burden of choice falls on you. Shopping is a personal choice, but information is power. Food labels have information - use it.

In the next chapter, you will learn how important the nutritional components of the staple foods are and their negative effects, if any.

CHAPTER EIGHT: STAPLES AS PART OF OUR HEALTHY DIET TODAY

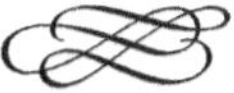

Have you ever been blindly accused of misconduct? How did that make you feel? Well, that is how staple foods feel. They have worked diligently over the years to fuel humanity, yet they face constant accusations by the same people without adequate grounds. Cereal grains, roots, and tubers have provided humanity's food bulk for centuries, and if history is anything to go by, all those generations cannot be wrong.

WHAT MAKES THEM GOOD?

There are numerous benefits we gain from the staples. The health of many people across the world would seriously suffer if the staple foods were to be eliminated. Hunger would sweep through all parts of the world and leave behind death and malnourished humans and animals. In addition to helping us stay alive and engage in different activities, staple foods are nutrient-rich. As we learned earlier, cereals are important sources of the vitamin B complex, carbohydrates, protein, iron, vitamin E, and some minerals.

Consumption of whole grains, roots, and tubers has various

health benefits, such as improving longevity, reduced chronic inflammation, lower risk of heart diseases, stroke, and type 2 diabetes mellitus, according to a study[1]carried out in 2015. Those foods should be the choice of those who are pursuing beach bodies, as they contribute to reduced belly fat and lower the risk of obesity. If you want a six-pack, they're for you. They also contribute to a lower risk of colon cancer. The fiber found in staples helps digestion and keeps us full for longer, preventing sugar cravings. Grains such as oats help to reduce blood sugar levels and are particularly beneficial for people suffering from insulin resistance, diabetes, or metabolic syndrome.

STARCH

Starch is a carbohydrate that naturally occurs in plants in varying amounts. The digestibility of starch is the main determinant of the available energy content of crops. However, not all the starch gets digested. Some pass through the digestive system unchanged and is called resistant starch, which acts as a soluble fiber. There are four types of starch. Type 1 resists digestion, as it is fixed within the fibrous cell walls of seeds, grains, and legumes. Type 2 occurs in some starchy foods like unripe bananas and raw potatoes. Type 3 forms after some starchy foods like rice and potatoes are cooked and cooled. Some digestible starches turn into resistant starches during cooling through retrogradation. Humans commonly manufacture type 4 starch through a chemical process.

Resistant starch improves insulin sensitivity, reduces appetite, lowers blood sugar levels, reduces the risk of colorectal cancer, and relieves various digestive disorders like diverticulitis, constipation, colitis, and Crohn's disease. Moreover, the higher the number of resistant starches in your food, the lower its calorie count, and the more full you will feel, making starchy foods ideal for weight management.

PROTEIN

Most staples do not have a high protein content, as found in other plants like legumes. However, they still form an important protein source for humans. Cereal grains account for about half of the protein requirements of human beings. Roots and tubers are not very protein-rich with 1-2 percent protein, in comparison to cereal grains, which contain 6-12 percent protein, although potatoes and yams are quite high in proteins. The protein quality of roots and tubers is, however, similar to that of animal proteins like eggs. Cereal proteins are an important component of the human diet - we eat about 16-45 grams per capita per day, and they represent roughly 70 percent of the available protein in some parts of the world.

Plant proteins have a lower content of essential amino acids due to the predominance of aleurins, or storage proteins, over enzymes, or cytoplasmic proteins. Enzymes have better nutritional quality than aleurins. Lower levels of essential amino acids help in preventing cardiovascular diseases by regulating cholesterol. Cereal proteins tend to be high in non-essential amino acids, which up-regulate glucagon and down-regulate insulin. As a result, they help to protect against chronic degenerative diseases, lower the risk factors for atherosclerosis, and retard cancer development. However, due to the low levels of proteins found in the staples, it is necessary to complement them with other rich sources like legumes.

CARBS AND COMPLEX CARBS

Carbohydrates are the body's main energy source. Since our staple foods are rich in carbs, they fuel the brain, muscles, kidneys, and nervous system. Fiber helps in digestion, keeps cholesterol levels in check, and keeps us full. Additionally, fiber acts as a molecular sieve that traps carcinogens, reducing the risk of diabetes, colon cancer, and heart diseases. The amount of vitamin B in roots and tubers is adequate to supplement other dietary sources. The B vitamins are involved in food oxidation and energy production

OTHER NUTRIENTS

Our bodies need other nutrients, such as vitamins and minerals, which vary from one crop to another. Roots and tubers are not rich in fat-soluble proteins, but Vitamin A is present in the form of beta-carotene in some crops like sweet potatoes. Vitamin C is found in considerable amounts in many of them. Cereal grains have B vitamins and vitamin E. The B vitamins thiamin, niacin, and riboflavin help in the release of energy from carbohydrates, fats, and proteins, and hence are important in metabolism. The other B vitamin in grains, folate, is crucial in the formation of red blood cells. Additionally, B vitamins help to maintain a healthy nervous system.

Other minerals found in staple foods include iron, which is important in the body's growth and development. The body uses iron in making myoglobin, a protein that supplies muscles with oxygen and hemoglobin, a protein that carries oxygen to all body parts. Iron is also necessary for the manufacture of hormones. Other minerals present in whole grains are selenium and magnesium. Selenium's role in the body is to protect cells from oxidation and to keep the immune system healthy. The body utilizes magnesium in the building of bones and the release of energy from muscles.

HOW THEY NEGATIVELY AFFECT US

Food is wonderful, but don't take its goodness for weakness. The high carbs found in staple foods can cause blood sugars to skyrocket when taken in large quantities, and could be especially harmful to people with diabetes. Moreover, overeating can cause digestive problems and discomfort through bloating. Grains contain antinutrients, which are substances that interfere with digestion. Wheat is particularly notorious for meting out punishment for the gluten-intolerant as well as causing digestive distress in others.

Refined staples are extremely unhealthy since they only have the high-carb, high-starch, and high-calorie endosperm with small amounts of protein. With the nutrients and fiber removed, they become empty calories that are easily absorbed by the body and broken down fast, causing rapid spikes in blood sugar. After spiking, blood sugar goes down just as fast, causing hunger and cravings and consequently overeating, weight gain, and obesity. Refined grains cause insulin resistance, heart diseases, and type 2 diabetes. The more you eat them, the hungrier you will get, and the more you will want to keep eating. While tasty, they can easily rope you in a cycle of unhealthy eating and cost you that beautiful body and your health.

CHAPTER SUMMARY

In addition to high levels of carbohydrates, staple foods are packed with proteins, vitamins, and minerals that are beneficial to our health. Overindulgence, particularly in refined foods, can cause a myriad of weight and health problems.

In the next chapter, you will learn how staples prevent or help to manage some ailments and diseases.

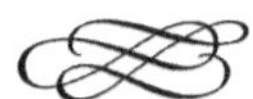

As we have seen in the previous chapter, staples contain nutrients that help either in the prevention or management of many ailments and diseases. Our ancestors used food as medicine. Can we do the same?

OBESITY

Do you know that obesity affects more people than malnutrition? While we are grateful for having more than enough to eat, it is also saddening to lose more than 2.8 million people each year to obesity. An obese person has excessive or abnormal body fat accumulation with a body mass index (BMI) of more than 30, which may impair health. Obesity is no vain concern, but a medical problem that requires intervention at the earliest stage before increasing the risk of other diseases like diabetes, heart diseases, and some cancers. It occurs due to a combination of inherited factors, diet, the environment, and physical activity.

While you may have limited ability to address the genetic, metabolic, behavioral, and hormonal influences on your body weight, you can prevent or manage obesity through diet and exercise. As long as you are not eating more calories than the body needs for daily activities, you cannot become obese. The increasing rate of obesity is due to the intake of foods loaded with calories and sedentary lifestyles. Staple foods are rich in dietary fiber that prevents overeating because fiber keeps you full for a long time. By eating less, you can either lose weight or prevent weight gain. Additionally, the consumption of unrefined staple foods daily lowers BMI and results in less body fat.

DIABETES

Diabetes is a condition that weakens the ability of the body to process blood sugar. If left unmanaged, diabetes can allow blood sugar to accumulate, which can cause complications like eye, nerve, and kidney damage, stroke, and cardiovascular disease. In 2014, over 422 million people had diabetes. For some people, the body does not produce insulin, causing type 1 diabetes or juvenile diabetes. For others, the body cells do not effectively respond to insulin, resulting in type 2 diabetes, which is strongly linked to obesity.

Eating complex carbohydrates rich in fiber, like brown rice, whole wheat, and quinoa, can help in the management of diabetes. Most unrefined staple foods have a low glycemic index and thus only cause a modest rise in blood sugar levels, which prevents the long-term complications associated with type 2 diabetes. Additionally, staple foods help in preventing obesity, which is a predisposing factor of type 2 diabetes. Furthermore, whole grains are linked to improved insulin sensitivity and lower fasting blood sugar levels. Magnesium found in whole grains helps in the metabolization of carbohydrates, which is tied to insulin sensitivity.

ALZHEIMER'S DISEASE AND DEMENTIA

Alzheimer's disease is a condition that causes brain cells to progressively degenerate and die. The main cause of dementia, a progressive decline in behavioral, thinking, and social skills that impairs one's ability to function, is Alzheimer's disease. Although strongly linked to age, Alzheimer's disease occurs due to a combination of lifestyle, environmental, and genetic factors that affect the brain. Alzheimer's disease and heart diseases share some of the common risk factors. Obesity, lack of exercise, smoking, high cholesterol, high blood pressure, and poorly controlled type 2 diabetes are some of them. Therefore, by ensuring a healthy diet of unrefined staple foods, you can prevent and control many of the risk factors like obesity, high cholesterol, and type 2 diabetes. The fiber and resistant starch in these foods prevent overeating, helps in controlling blood sugar and cholesterol levels, and promotes a healthy heart.

OSTEOPOROSIS

Imagine having bones so weak and brittle that they break from coughing or even bending. Bones are living tissues, and they get replaced when they break down. However, in some instances, the supply does not keep up with the demand. The body is not able to manufacture new ones fast enough to replace those that break down. No one wants to be in such a situation. The good news is that weight-bearing exercises and a healthy diet can help in the prevention of bone loss and strengthen weak bones. Staple foods can help, as they provide a healthy source of nutrients. Some of the risk factors of osteoporosis include hormone levels, dietary factors like low calcium intake, gastrointestinal surgery, and eating disorders. Medical conditions such as inflammatory bowel disease, celiac disease, cancer, kidney or liver disease, and poor lifestyle choices like alcohol and tobacco use are also risk factors.

Being either overweight or underweight increases the risk of fractures. By eating unrefined staple foods, you can maintain appropriate body weight. Additionally, the high amount of fiber found in staples can help to reduce the risk of inflammatory bowel disease and some cancers. However, some staples like wheat, rye, and barley contain gluten, which causes celiac disease in some people. Other staples like roots and tubers, millet, quinoa, maize, and rice can provide the necessary nutrients without the risk of celiac disease.

HIGH CHOLESTEROL AND HIGH BLOOD PRESSURE

The staples help in the prevention and management of both high cholesterol and high blood pressure. Eating whole grains provides the body with high amounts of fiber, which lowers cholesterol levels and keeps you feeling full for long. By reducing cholesterol level, you fight off high blood pressure, since arteries are not restricted and blood can flow freely. Additionally, unrefined staples help in reaching and maintaining a healthy weight that lowers blood pressure. Staples also help to cut sugar out of the diet by keeping you full, preventing sugar cravings and the need to snack.

CORONARY ARTERY DISEASE (ISCHEMIC HEART DISEASE)

As the name suggests, ischemic heart disease stems from the coronary arteries, the blood vessels that supply blood and oxygen to the heart. Ischemia is the inadequate supply of blood to a body part caused by the blockage of the vessels supplying that area. If you have been to a farm with drip irrigators, you may have come across blocked lines. While the other crops thrive, those supplied by the blocked lines wither away. The principle is similar. Coronary Heart Disease (CHD) is a result of cholesterol building up on the walls of coronary arteries and creating plaque. The arteries then become narrow, reducing blood flow. In some instances, a clot occurs that obstructs blood flow, causing severe health problems like heart attacks.

Unlike the repairable drip line, CHD has no cure. However,

it is not all grim. The condition is manageable through making healthy lifestyle changes like a healthy diet, exercise, and not smoking. Moreover, the risk factors of CHD like obesity, hypertension, high cholesterol, and type 2 diabetes can be reduced through the intake of unrefined staples. Whole grains, roots, and tubers contain a high number of resistant carbohydrates hence high fiber content, bound antioxidants, and nutrients. As such, they help in reducing blood pressure, fostering weight loss, and lowering blood sugar, all of which help in managing CHD.

STROKE

Stroke is a dangerous cousin to CHD. Like CHD, strokes are caused by an interruption or reduced supply of nutrients and oxygen, but this time to part of the brain. The disruption causes brain cells to start dying in a matter of minutes. A stroke that results from a blocked artery is called an ischemic stroke, while a hemorrhagic stroke occurs from a blood vessel's leak or a burst. Dietary fiber in staples can help prevent strokes by addressing some of the risk factors, such as obesity or overweight, high blood pressure, high cholesterol, diabetes, and cardiovascular disease. Furthermore, taking unrefined staple foods instead of refined foods helps to prevent high cholesterol levels and thus prevent ischemia. Reducing blood pressure is also crucial in preventing vessels from leaking or bursting.

CHRONIC LOWER RESPIRATORY INFECTIONS

Chronic lower respiratory infections affect the lungs or below the voice box and encompass COPD (Chronic Obstructive Pulmonary Disease), chronic bronchitis, emphysema, asthma, occupational lung disease, and pulmonary hypertension. They are mainly characterized by dyspnea (shortness of breath) due to an obstructed airway. The World Health Organization estimates that 65 million people suffer from moderate to severe COPD.

While the predominant risk factor is smoking, environmental factors, infections, occupational hazards, and exposure to second-hand smoke also play a role.

You could be wondering how breathing and eating could be related. Remember, we are a mass of interrelated networks - if one part of you gets hurt, the rest of the body always seems to support the hurt part. Everything within us is connected. When you eat, food undergoes metabolism to become the fuel that the body can use. The metabolism process uses food and oxygen as the inputs and produces carbon dioxide and energy as the outputs. Your body takes in oxygen and breathes out carbon dioxide. Therefore, a well-balanced diet allows you to breathe easy, literally. Research[1] has shown that eating healthy food, such as whole grains and nuts that are rich in polyunsaturated fats, lowers the risk of COPD by promoting a well-functioning lung. The diet should include complex carbohydrates and 20-30 grams of fiber per day, which can be found in staple foods, and few simple sugars. Besides, lower respiratory disorders affect under-weight people disproportionately, and staple foods can help in healthy weight gain.

CANCERS

The world today is grappling with over 100 menacing cancers that torture the peace out of the human body. Cancer refers to abnormal cells growing uncontrollably in the body and edging out the normal cells. Cancer cells are like humans: determined to expand and dominate. There are over 100 different types of cancer, each with its own personality. Some grow slowly, others spread quickly, and while many respond to treatment, others are adamant and refuse to budge. However, humans' stronger determination has ensured that cancer is more manageable now than ever before. Many people overcome cancer to lead a healthy life, and age-old staples are always there to help.

Researchers have indicated that a healthy diet can help in the prevention of 30-50 percent of all cancers. That is not all. Proper nutrition is vital in treating as well as coping with cancer. On the other hand, consumption of refined carbs and sugars increases the risk of breast, colorectal, and stomach cancers. Alongside infection and smoking, obesity is the most significant risk factor, increasing the risk of thirteen types of cancer. By now, you are well-informed on managing obesity by eating staple foods. What you should now know is that a plant-based diet can reduce the risk of developing or succumbing to cancer. Whole grains are particularly well-suited for prevention against cancer.

DEHYDRATION DUE TO DIARRHEAL DISEASE

Losing a child can be unbearably distressing and torturing, at the least. Now, consider that each year, over 525,000 parents of children under five go through this agony due to diarrhea. To add insult to injury, diarrheal disease is both preventable and treatable. It leaves the body dehydrated as it causes the passage of more than three liquid stools a day, leaving the body without the salts and water necessary for survival. Diarrhea is the result of an intestinal tract infection that could be due to viral, bacterial, or parasitic organisms. Additionally, children who succumb to diarrhea, in most cases, suffer from malnutrition. Malnutrition increases their vulnerability to diarrhea, which in turn worsens malnutrition. Staples help in providing nutrient-rich sources of food that are accessible and affordable. Besides being rich in energy, staples contain proteins and other minerals that can help keep both hunger and malnutrition away. Moreover, many roots and tubers contain a high percentage of water that can help hydrate the affected children while also providing food. Their leaves are also good sources of vitamins and iron. Children need access to healthy and nutrient-rich foods like staples.

TUBERCULOSIS (TB)

Tuberculosis claimed about 1.5 million people in 2018, with 10 million infected worldwide. TB is an airborne bacterial infection caused by Mycobacterium tuberculosis that affects the lungs. The good news is that TB is not only preventable but also curable. A TB patient needs to have a healthy diet with essential nutrients, including carbohydrates, proteins, vitamins, minerals, fats, and water. In particular, the food should have high energy without high volume. Insufficient nutrition is a risk factor for TB and also weakens the ability of the body to fight it, leaving the person susceptible to reinfection or relapse. High-energy foods are packed with nutrients to build a strong immunity that helps to fight off TB.

ANXIETY

We have all been anxious before tests, results, interviews, or even a date. That is normal and healthy. What if you were extremely anxious all the time? Constantly filled with fear, worry and apprehension? Wouldn't you be concerned? You could and should, because anxiety disorders exist. They can change how you process emotions and behave to the extent of causing physical symptoms like nausea and increased blood pressure. Maintaining a healthy diet, drinking adequate water, and limiting caffeine and alcohol can help in relieving anxiety. Eating complex carbohydrates, abundantly found in staples, helps in achieving a more stable blood sugar level, which is calming. Additionally, studies found that magnesium, found in whole grains, helps one to feel calm.

INSOMNIA

We have seen that staples help in relieving anxiety, but do you know that they are also instrumental in dealing with insomnia?

Have you ever stayed awake when the world around you was snoring away? Imagine enduring that three or more times a week for extended periods. Well, 30 percent of the population has difficulties falling or staying asleep or wakes up too early and can't sleep again. The major causes of insomnia include stress, poor sleep habits, and work or travel schedules, mainly when jobs cover different time zones. Believe it or not, overeating, particularly in the evening, is a common cause of insomnia. We should thank our ancestors for making food so readily available to us that it now costs us our sleep.

Diet influences sleep quality. Foods containing refined carbohydrates and added sugars, like white rice, white bread, and soda, are strongly linked to a high risk of insomnia. A quick rise in blood sugar prompts the body to release insulin, which helps to lower it, causing the release of cortisol and adrenaline that may cause sleep interferences. Therefore, having meals with staple foods, such as whole grains and tubers, can help with sleep because they do not cause sudden spikes in blood sugar levels. Moreover, they keep you full for longer so you do not have to wake up because of hunger.

CHAPTER SUMMARY

In this chapter, you have learned that food is medicine. Eating a healthy diet is vital in maintaining health. Staple foods help in preventing infections and boosting immunity so that the body can fight off existing infections. Additionally, good food taken in appropriate portions can help with relaxing the mind and promoting a healthy state of mind.

Since we have talked extensively about carbohydrates, you get a bonus chapter that will help increase your understanding of them. Hopefully, you can establish a beautiful and beneficial relationship with them.

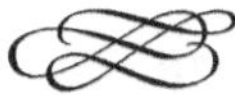

WHAT IS CARBOHYDRATE?

A carbohydrate, also called a saccharide, is a biological molecule made up of carbon, hydrogen, and oxygen atoms. Biomolecules are any of the numerous substances produced by cells and living organisms. The main types of biomolecules are carbohydrates, nucleic acids, lipids, and proteins. Of these, carbohydrates are the most abundant. Carbs are made up of two essential compounds: aldehydes and ketones. Aldehydes have a carbon-oxygen double bond attached to a hydrogen atom, while ketones lack the hydrogen atom. The three types of carbohydrates are monosaccharides, disaccharides, and polysaccharides.

Simply, carbohydrates are naturally occurring starches, fiber, and sugars that are broken down by the body into glucose for feeding the cells. Sugar is a simple carb, while fiber and starch are complex carbs. Carbohydrates are one of the main classes of food alongside vitamins and proteins and the primary source of energy.

COMPLEX CARBOHYDRATES

A complex carbohydrate is made up of long and complex sugar molecules threaded together in long and complex chains. Also known as polysaccharides or oligosaccharides, these carbohydrates take longer to digest. Complex carbohydrates may contain vitamins, minerals, and fiber, which the body takes a long time to digest. Examples include whole grain like brown rice, oatmeal, bulgur, whole-grain barley, and wild rice. Other complex carbohydrates include grains like buckwheat and quinoa, non-starchy vegetables like zucchini, starchy staples like corn and sweet potatoes, and legumes like chickpeas and kidney beans.

IMPORTANCE OF CARBOHYDRATES

The primary function of carbs is to provide energy for the body. Once ingested, carbohydrates are broken down through digestion into glucose, which enters the bloodstream. The glucose is used by cells to produce adenosine triphosphate, or ATP, used as fuel for various metabolic tasks. If the amount of glucose in the body exceeds its current needs, the extra, called glycogen, is stored mainly in muscles and liver for later use. Once the body's glycogen stores are full, the excess is stored as fat. Carbohydrates also help in the preservation of muscles by providing glucose energy for the brain and thus prevent the breakdown of muscles. The brain requires energy, even during starvation. If there is no glucose for use, the body begins to break down muscles, which we need in order to move. Therefore, during starvation, a few carbs go a long way in ensuring you can move again.

Carbohydrates also promote proper digestion, since they contain fiber which is not broken down into glucose. Fiber helps in bowel movement and protects against digestive tract diseases. Carbohydrates, particularly complex carbs, help in managing blood sugar levels and promoting a healthy heart. Fiber helps in delaying carbs' absorption in the digestive tract, preventing sugar spikes after a meal. Moreover, fiber binds to bile acids in the small intestines and prevents their reabsorption. The liver, therefore, has to use cholesterol to make more bile acids, thus reducing cholesterol in the body.

THE OVERALL ROLE OF CARBS IN PHYSICAL AND MENTAL HEALTH

Carbohydrates serve several vital functions in the body, the most important being the supply of energy for daily tasks. They are the main source of fuel for the brain, an organ with high energy demand. Also, fiber promotes a healthy digestive tract and lowers the risk of diverticular diseases. Additionally, fiber helps in reducing the risk of diabetes and heart disease by maintaining appropriate blood sugar and cholesterol levels. Complex carbohydrates are also significant in relieving anxiety and promoting good sleep. In essence, carbs are an essential part of a healthy diet and are crucial in the prevention and management of many diseases. They boost immunity and promote overall good health.

HARMFUL CARBS

Taking too much of anything turns it from useful to poisonous. While carbs are good sources of energy, they can also be harmful when taken in large quantities. Take sugary drinks, for example. Sugar is a natural part of carbohydrates. However, the processed sugar added to drinks is one of the most horrible ingredients in refined foods today. Liquid calories do not register as food in the brain, and hence, you can easily keep going. In large amounts, sugar can cause insulin resistance and fatty liver disease. Furthermore, sugary drinks can easily make you fat and obese.

Another culprit is white bread. We love white bread for its pleasant taste, despite knowing that it is not a healthy option. White flour is made from grains whose germ and bran have been removed, only leaving the endosperm. In the absence of vitamins, fiber, and minerals, the endosperm only provides easily digestible carbohydrates. Products made with refined flours can lead to obesity, diabetes, and heart disease. Moreover, most types of bread have added sugars that further increase calories.

In some parts of the world, breakfast and cereals go together. Breakfast cereals are processed using different types of grains like oats, corn, rice, and wheat. They all purport to be healthy, and they would be, except that they are high in added sugar. Taken in high amounts, they put you at risk of obesity, diabetes, and heart diseases. You should avoid sweetened cereals and opt for those low in sugar and high in fiber. However, it may be difficult to tell which ones are legit. Therefore, it may be better to make such foods like porridge. Oat porridge is fast and easy to make.

Potato chips and French fries should be taken in minimal quantities, if at all. We learned earlier that the potato is healthy. However, when baked, fried, or roasted, they may have many acrylamides, which are carcinogenic substances. They also tend to be calorie-dense and easy to overeat, contributing to excessive weight gain.

Also, skip dessert. The delicious cakes and pastries are only good to look at. How many only eat a small piece of cake? The rest eat only a tiny piece at a time until it is gone. Next time you eye the dessert, remember that most of them are packed with added sugars and refined flours. In addition to being fattening, they expose you to the risk of developing diabetes and heart diseases. They don't make your teeth happy, either.

FOODS THAT ACCOMPANY CARBS FOR A HEALTHY BODY

Your body needs a well-balanced diet to operate optimally. In addition to carbohydrates, you need to ensure that you eat proteins, vitamins, and minerals. You can obtain proteins from both plant and animal sources, including seafood, eggs, legumes, beef, dairy products, poultry, and pork. In addition to providing proteins, they also help to keep you full. You should take care to eat the right amount.

Vitamins are essential in boosting our immunity. They are also great accompaniments to carbs. You can get different vitamins from a wide range of foods such as vegetables, almonds, milk, vegetable oils, and eggs. Minerals are also essential additions to the diet. They include calcium obtained from dark leafy greens and dairy products. Sources of chromium include beef, fish, broccoli, grape juice, and turkey. Organic meats like kidney and liver, avocadoes, seafood, and sunflower seeds are some of the foods rich in copper. Iron is also an important mineral that you can get from such foods as leafy greens, shellfish, soy foods, red meat, and eggs.

Carbs can get lonely and would appreciate some company. Serve them with some vegetables, meats, legumes, seafood, nuts, fruits, and oils. Make your plate colorful and balanced. You will not only enjoy eating, but also reap the full benefits of a healthy diet. Top it all up with water - it is life!

WHICH FOODS ARE RICH IN CARBOHYDRATES?

Since carbohydrates are the largest food group and primary providers of energy, they are widely found in foods around us. Grains are carb-rich and include wheat, rice, millet, maize, barley, rye, and sorghum. Legumes such as beans, peas, and cowpeas are rich not only in proteins but also in carbohydrates. Most people associate dairy with calcium and proteins, but dairy products like yogurt, milk, and ice cream are also rich in carbs. Roots and tubers like potatoes, cassava, sweet potatoes, and yams are relevant sources of carbohydrates. The sweetness in fruits which makes them highly palatable, is due to sugars, which are carbohydrates. Some dangerous sources of carbs are sugary sweets like soda, cookies, and candy. Let me repeat: please skip dessert. Moderation hardly works there.

CHAPTER SUMMARY

Now you have a clear understanding that carbs are natural sugars, starches, and fibers that fuel humanity. Complex carbohydrates are best to eat as they contain high amounts of fiber. Also, you should avoid refined carbohydrates, the ones that give the others a bad name. Enjoy your carbs in moderation and add proteins, vitamins, and minerals to make a delicious and healthy meal.

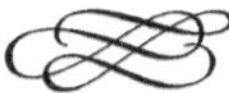

WHAT IS GLUTEN?

The elastic and chewy texture that occurs in the dough is a result of gluten. Before we embark on the reason gluten is now famous, let us look at what it is. Gluten is a family of storage proteins, known as prolamins, which naturally occur in cereal grains like wheat, barley, spelt, and rye. There are two main proteins in gluten; gliadin and glutenin.

When heated, gluten proteins form an elastic network that is stretchable and can trap gas allowing for rising, optimal leavening and moisture maintenance. We are then able to bake bread and get a satisfying texture. Due to these characteristics, gluten is used as an additive for texture improvement and moisture retention in some processed foods.

FOODS HIGH IN GLUTEN

Many of the cereal grains contain gluten. However, wheat takes the gold medal here and is commonly associated with gluten. Many people think only wheat has gluten and opting for other grains means eating gluten-free. That is not true. Let us look at some of the gluten-containing foods as well as their products.

On top of the list is wheat, including its various varieties and derivatives like spelt, farina, durum, wheat berries, semolina, graham, and Ferro. Others like rye, triticale, barley, brewer's yeast, and malt in all its forms also contain gluten.

In essence, all products derived from any of the foods listed above also contain gluten. Things like noodles, pasta, bread, pastries, crackers, breakfast cereals, tortillas, beer, and baked goods all contain gluten. Your breakfast possibly includes foods rich in gluten like pancakes, French toast, waffles, and cookies. Since gluten is used as an additive, it may be difficult to tell for sure which products contain gluten. For example, gluten lurks in frozen vegetables, sauces, supplements, medicine, and even some toothpaste.

WHY DO PEOPLE GO GLUTEN-FREE?

You are most likely wondering what the hula boo is about gluten. You eat all those foods every day, and you are still alive and full of energy. All of a sudden, it seems everyone has gone gluten-free. The supermarkets' aisles are screaming gluten-free, and your favorite restaurant is also offering gluten-free options. The bread you have eaten daily for years is now bad because it contains gluten, a natural protein.

People are switching to gluten-free foods to aid weight loss, increase energy, feel healthier, and treat conditions like autism. Despite the gluten-free craze, most people are not affected by gluten in any way. Thus, going gluten-free may simply be a waste of money and a limit to variety in their diet. However, some people are gluten-intolerant. They develop adverse reactions to even small amounts of gluten. People suffering from celiac disease are particularly intolerant to as little as 50 milligrams of gluten, which can trigger an immune response that causes damages to the gastrointestinal lining, inflames in the small intestines, and reduce the efficiency of the body in absorbing nutrients.

Even if you do not react adversely to gluten, you can opt to go gluten-free since gluten can be inflammatory and cause or exacerbate joint pains, swelling, and conditions like arthritis. Additionally, those who have thyroid problems may benefit from a gluten-free diet as it has been shown to reduce antibodies linked to autoimmune thyroid disease.

Gluten- dense products like bread are not considered a necessary part of diet by many people. In fact, most fad diets eliminate them, and hence, people go gluten-free for perceived benefits like weight loss and better health. Additionally, many people, about 13% of humanity, suffer from sensitivities to gluten. After consuming food products with gluten, they may suffer from stomach upsets, skin problems, brain fog, and irregular bowel movements.

WHICH FOODS TO AVOID IF YOU HAVE A GLUTEN INTOLERANCE?

Not everyone experiences much discomfort from gluten. Some of us wolf down slices of bread, pancakes, and crackers with only the discomfort of being too full – for a while. However, for those sensitive and intolerant to gluten, the price is much higher. They, therefore, have to ensure that the foods they take do not contain any gluten.

If you are gluten intolerant, you need to stay away from mother wheat and all her children. To be safe, include the entire generation. That means wheat, its bread, whether white, whole wheat, brown, or flatbread. Included also in this list are pancakes, tortillas, pasta, noodles, and wheat crackers. In essence, anything that is derived from wheat is a no-go zone. Other grains to avoid include rye, barley, spelt, Kamut, triticale, farina, farro, wheat berries, and couscous. All products that contain any derivatives of these grains also contain gluten and are best to avoid.

While there are some gluten-free bread, wraps, and crackers, you need to choose cautiously since many of them contain gluten. Therefore, it is best to check the list of ingredients closely. Do not be fooled by the big signs for healthy versions. Before making any purchase, your work is to check the list of ingredients keenly and ensure the product does not contain anything that would have gluten.

You also need to be careful before taking certain condiments. They are not the ideal candidates for gluten, but many of them are made with ingredients containing gluten or it is used as an additive. These include barbecue sauce, marinades, soy sauce, ketchup, cream sauces, malt vinegar, gravy mixes, and salad dressings. Smile, it is not all gloom. You can purchase those certified to be gluten-free or simply make your own at home.

If you have a sour relationship with gluten, then you need to stay away from the bakery. Most baked goods use wheat flour or other grains containing gluten. Things like cakes, cookies, doughnuts, muffins, and pastries need to stay far from your mouth. You may also not enjoy some common snacks like granola bars, pretzels, chips, snack mixes, energy bars, and candy bars. Unfortunately, it is not just what you eat but also what you drink. Some beverages like beer, drink mixes, premade coffee, wine, and chocolate milk may contain gluten.

As a cautionary measure, you have to read food labels keenly or buy certified gluten-free products. Alternatively, you can grow or make much of the food items as possible.

HOW DO YOU KNOW IF GLUTEN IS AN IRRITANT FOR YOU?

You are probably wondering if gluten affects you. Trying to think back to that one time you felt bloated after a meal and beginning to point fingers at gluten. Don't be too fast. The effect of gluten on people's health matters; while it doesn't affect some, others are mildly irritated, while for others, it comes with adverse effects.

One of the most common symptoms of gluten irritability is bloating, where you have a swollen stomach or feel gassy. As high as 87% of people with gluten sensitivity experience bloating. In addition to bloating, if you are gluten sensitive, you could experience constipation, diarrhea, or smelly feces. Other symptoms include abdominal pains, headaches, brain fog, and feeling tired, even when all you have done is eat. Some people may also experience skin problems such as dermatitis herpetiformis, which manifests celiac disease. Joint pains and numbness are also part of the common symptoms of gluten irritability.

Interestingly, you can get anxiety and autoimmune diseases. You could also get depression courtesy of gluten. Yes, this is due to abnormal levels of serotonin. Serotonin is a happiness hormone, and its low levels can cause one to get depressed. Gluten could make you depressed through the production of gluten exorphins during digestion that may interfere with the efficient running of the central nervous system, increasing the risk of depression. Additionally, changes in the gut's microbiota to include more harmful bacteria than beneficial ones raise the risk of depression.

The struggle for weight loss is universal. Most of us have been on one diet or another. However, unexpected weight loss is a cause for concern. For people with gluten intolerance, it could be a sign of celiac disease.

MEDICAL CONDITIONS WHICH CAN CAUSE ONE TO HAVE A GLUTEN-FREE DIET

Celiac Disease-The main medical condition that calls for a gluten-free diet is Celiac disease, which is a chronic disorder of the digestive system. This disease results from an immune reaction to the gluten protein, gliadin that causes the inflammation and damage of a person's small intestines' inner lining. The result is malabsorption of nutrients and minerals. Symptoms include weight loss, fatigue, and chronic diarrhea. In some cases, anemia is the only symptom and is mainly diagnosed later on in life. Approximately one person in 141 Americans has celiac disease. If you suffer from a celiac disease, you will likely end up with malnutrition due to poor absorption of minerals and nutrients.

Non-celiac gluten sensitivity-Unfortunately the list of conditions associated with gluten does not stop with celiac disease. Some people have gluten sensitivity, not necessarily a celiac disease, but a condition referred to as NCGS (Non-celiac gluten sensitivity). Gluten sensitivity, however, is the main cause of Celiac Disease. NCGS describes a condition where a person does not have a wheat allergy or celiac disease but displays extra-intestinal symptoms, intestinal symptoms, or both related to the consumption of grains containing products, with visible improvements upon withdrawal. NCGS has no biomarkers and is often wrongly interpreted as an irritable bowel movement. Diagnosis requires the exclusion of wheat allergy and celiac disease. NCGS is the most common ailment linked to gluten, with a prevalence rate of between 0.5% and 13%.

Dermatitis Herpetiformis (DH)-also called Duhring's disease, is an itchy and bumpy skin rash that commonly affects people with celiac disease. It causes blisters that resemble herpes but occur as a result of gluten sensitivity.

Gluten Ataxia- Although there is yet to be a clear explanation of how gluten ataxia occurs, it is thought to result from postulated antibodies that affect the cerebellum causing the damage. In many cases, celiac disease antibodies tend to be more than the normal population. For Gluten Ataxia, while a gluten-free diet could be helpful, sometimes the cerebellum damage is irreversible and causes degeneration and atrophy.

If you have any of these conditions, it is best to avoid gluten. Going gluten-free remains the best way of managing medical conditions related to the intake of products containing gluten.

WHAT FOODS SHOULD A GLUTEN-FREE DIET CONTAIN?

You may want to go gluten-free for one reason or the other. Looking back at the list of what to avoid, it may seem like there is typically nothing left to eat. Relax, Mother Nature is extremely generous. Besides, she knew some of her children would not deal well with gluten.

There are other grains you can eat. These include brown rice, sorghum, millet, amaranth, quinoa, wild rice. Tapioca, and oats. However, in many cases, oats are transported and processed with equipment that is shared with wheat. They, therefore, are likely to contain some gluten. If you would like to eat oats, you must look for those certified as being gluten-free. You also have the choice of tubers like arrowroots, potatoes, sweet potatoes, and yams.

Fresh vegetables and fruits naturally do not contain gluten. You can enjoy these while still succulent. Once processed, they may contain gluten that is used as a thickener or for flavoring. Pile up your plate with carrots, onions, green beans, greens, mushrooms, and berries. Any fresh fruit or vegetable that tickles your fancy is safe.

For proteins, you can relax – a bit. You have a wide variety of nuts, seeds, legumes, poultry, seafood, red meat, and traditional soy foods. In essence, proteins in their natural state are gluten-free. However, the surety disappears with processing. You have to be careful with processed meats, meat substitutes, ground meats, meat mixed with sauces, cold cuts, and those microwave dinners we love to make on those days that we can barely lift a finger.

Bring out the dairy! Being gluten intolerant is not being lactose intolerant. Enjoy a glass of milk or yogurt, spread the cheese, ghee, and butter, and don't forget to whip some cream. You, however, need to double-check the flavored varieties, processed cheese, and ice cream. Stay clear of malted milk.

Fats and Oils- These are gluten-free. You can use olive oil, avocado oil, seed and vegetable oil, coconut oil, butter, or ghee. Take precautions with cooking sprays and spiced/flavored oil.

You can drink too. In addition to water, you have 100% fruit juices, tea, coffee, sports drinks, energy drinks, soda, lemonade, and some alcoholic drinks made from gluten-free grains.

Some spices and condiments like tamari, white, apple cider, distilled vinegar, and coconut amino are safe. You can also use fresh herbs and make your condiments at home to ensure they are gluten-free.

OATS AND AVENIN

There exists a major debate on whether oats should be part of a gluten-free diet or not. While oats in their pure form do not contain gluten, their processing and transport mainly occur in the same places as many gluten-containing grains like wheat and, thus, tend to be contaminated. Additionally, oats contain a protein whose chemical structure is similar to gluten called avenin. Due to their similarity, some people with celiac disease also react to avenin. However, only a small percentage, one in ten people, experience an immune reaction. Mild symptoms like stomach pain, bloating, and diarrhea are more common.

If you have celiac disease, you do not necessarily need to avoid avenin since the likelihood of having a severe reaction is very low. Besides, oats provide much-needed fiber for the body and help with digestive problems.

WHEAT ALLERGY

Many people are allergic to grains, and wheat seems to notoriously cross many people the wrong way. A wheat allergy develops when the immune system gets sensitive and overreacts to wheat that typically does not affect most people. Once exposed to wheat, the person develops symptoms like hives, headaches, asthma, runny nose, stomach cramps, indigestion, nausea, or diarrhea.

Wheat allergy is not synonymous with gluten intolerance. People with wheat allergy can eat other gluten-containing cereals. Avoiding wheat and its products is your best bet when managing a wheat allergy.

GLUTEN-FREE LABELING

With the increasing popularity of a gluten-free diet, manufacturers are now labeling products as gluten-free. The beauty is that many gluten-sensitive people now have an easy time picking ideal products, while on the other hand, manufacturers are promoting sales. The gluten-free label is a voluntary claim; however, the FDA (Food and Drug Administration) rule holds manufacturers responsible for using the label. The FDA expects manufacturers to lay an accurate claim that is not misleading in any manner and one that complies with all the FDA requirements.

Specifically, any food labeled as being 'gluten-free', 'without gluten', 'no-gluten', or 'free of gluten' must contain fewer than 20 ppm (parts per million) of gluten, the lowest reliably detectable level. Additionally, any food that contains any type of rye, barley, wheat or a crossbreed of either cannot be labelled as gluten-free. Neither can any ingredients derived from these grains without their processing to remove gluten. If the grains undergo processing to remove gluten, the resulting food must contain gluten levels of 20 ppm or below.

Since August 2014, manufacturers have had to comply with the FDA regulations on gluten-free labeling. You need to note that not all products are labeled as gluten-free, even when they meet the required conditions. For instance, water is gluten-free, but you will hardly come across any brand labeled as such.

The FDA's gluten-free labeling regulations apply to all foods and beverages except for certain egg products, poultry, and meat regulated by the USDA and most alcoholic beverages regulated by the Department of Treasury's Alcohol and Tobacco Tax and Trade Bureau.

GLUTEN AND HEALTH BENEFITS

A lot has been said about gluten, and like an accused person who is confident in his innocence, it quietly watches as people tarnish its name. Gluten has been a natural part of our diet for millions of years, yet the modern man feels that letting gluten into their body is wrong. Media reports and catchy headlines have not made life easy for gluten. They say a gluten-free diet is a way to avoid brain fog, bloating, inflammation, and heart diseases. Gluten, away from all the allegations, offers major health benefits.

Reduced risk of type 2 diabetes: According to the American Heart Association in 2017, a study of 199,794 people reported that those who ate gluten had a 13% lower risk of developing type 2 diabetes.

Lower risk of heart diseases: Gluten has been cited as a contributing factor to heart diseases, which is far from the truth. A 25-year study by Harvard School of Public Health involving more than 100,000 participants did not find any link between the long-term consumption of gluten and a high risk of heart diseases. Conversely, it established that those with a high gluten intake also had a much lower risk of heart diseases. Thus, those without gluten intolerance should increase their intake of gluten-containing grains.

Fewer calories: the nutritional composition of gluten-containing foods includes fewer calories than gluten-free counterparts. Gluten-free diets tend to have considerably more protein, calories, sugar, and saturated fatty acids. For a trimmer body and better health, it is best to include gluten-containing grains in your diet.

Decreased risk of colorectal cancer: Whole grains, including those containing gluten, contain high amounts of fiber that help in the prevention of diseases. They also help reduce the risk of colorectal cancer by 17% per 90 grams of whole grains consumed in a day. Besides, gluten acts as a prebiotic that feeds the beneficial bacteria in the body. A healthy body needs these bacteria in the gut. Changes in their numbers and activity are linked to gastrointestinal diseases such as irritable bowel syndrome, inflammatory bowel disease, and colorectal cancer. Therefore, a portion of whole grains a day, keeps things moving and sickness away.

However, if you are gluten intolerant, it would be wise and safe to keep away from gluten. However, you may need to put in the effort to ensure that you do not miss out on the health benefits associated with gluten by designing your diet in a manner that allows you to get all the necessary nutrients.

CHAPTER SUMMARY

Gluten is a naturally occurring protein found in grains like wheat, rye, and barley. Unfortunately, not everyone reacts well to gluten, and some may have intolerances that cause various symptoms like bloating, diarrhea, stomach pains, skin problems, brain fog, and joint pains, among others. More serious effects include celiac disease that affects about 1% of the population. Gluten, however, has numerous health benefits, especially due to its high fiber content. You may have heard of its negatives, but gluten helps lower the risk of type 2 diabetes, heart diseases, and colorectal cancer. Not unless gluten negatively affects you, include it in your diet. Nature gave us grains to fuel and heal us.

The bad reputation associated with staple foods does not originate from their natural abilities. Whole grains are immensely healthy and known for many health benefits. It is our choice to keep refining them, thus stripping them of their nutrients, and consistently ingest them that is the problem. Since we do not want to face ourselves, we blame our unhealthy habits on the foods that fuel the world.

Our love for beauty and taste has overridden our self-respect. We would rather eat delicious but empty calories than have good health. We forget that nature has a solution for our taste buds. Instead of taking out all the goodness from our staple foods, let us embrace nature and spice things up! There are many spices and herbs that we can use to improve the taste of food that does not appeal to us. The inclusion of different foods in varied colors to our diet can also improve its appearance. Let's get creative - we are humans!

Lastly, let us be ambassadors of the goodness of our age-old staple foods. They are not only energy-giving foods but also preventive and curative medicine. They have medicated humanity over the years and will continue to do so if we take them in the right proportion and mixed with other foods to provide a good balance. Furthermore, we need to embrace eating whole staple foods as much as possible to enjoy their full nature-intended benefits. After all, they are our heritage from our ancestors, meant to heal us and ensure we live healthy, wealthy, and full lives.

SOURCES

American Cancer Society (2020). Cancer Basics. https://www.cancer.org/cancer/cancer-basics.html

American Lung Association (2020). Nutrition and COPD. https://www.lung.org/lung-health-diseases/lung-disease-lookup/copd/living-with-copd/nutrition

Ancient Civilizations World (2017).Ancient Civilizations: Food and Eating. https://ancientcivilizationsworld.com/food/

Archaeology Organization (2020). Earliest Spears. https://www.archaeology.org/issues/81-1303/trenches/523-south-africa-earliest-spears

Barbara Pickersgill, Domestication of Plants in the Americas: Insights from Mendelian and Molecular Genetics, Annals of Botany, Volume 100, Issue 5, October 2007, Pages 925–940, https://doi.org/10.1093/aob/mcm193

BBC Future (2020). The past, present and future of food.

https://www.bbc.com/future/article/20161104-the-past-present-and-future-of-the-food

Burney, P., Perez-Padilla, R., Marks, G., Wong, G., Bateman, E., & Jarvis, D. (2017). Chronic lower respiratory tract diseases. In Cardiovascular, Respiratory, and Related Disorders. 3rd edition. The International Bank for Reconstruction and Development/The World Bank.

Cohut, M (2019). How diet may lead to insomnia. Medical News Today. https://www.medicalnewstoday.com/articles/327302

Crops of the Early Farmers ." Ancient Europe, 8000 B.C. to A.D. 1000: Encyclopedia of the Barbarian World. . Retrieved August 04, 2020 from Encyclopedia.com: https://www.encyclopedia.com/humanities/encyclopedias-almanacs-transcripts-and-maps/crops-early-farmers

Davis, C (2020). Cancer. Medicinenet. https://www.medicinenet.com/cancer/article.htm

Duvall,Z (2019). Farmers are Feeding our Growing Economies Early Agriculture and the Rise of Civilization ." Science and Its Times: Understanding the Social Significance of Scientific Discovery. . Retrieved August 03, 2020 from Encyclopedia.com: https://www.encyclopedia.com/science/encyclopedias-almanacs-transcripts-and-maps/early-agriculture-and-rise-civilization
Early diet.http://gby.huji.ac.il/

Eggum, B. O. (1977). Nutritional aspects of cereal proteins. In Genetic diversity in plants (pp. 349-369). Springer, Boston, MA.

FAO, IFAD, UNICEF, WFP, WHO. (2019). The state of food security and nutrition in the world 2019: safeguarding against economic slowdowns and downturns. http://www.fao.org/state-of-food-security-nutrition

Felman, A (2020). What to know about Anxiety. Medical News Today. https://www.medicalnewstoday.com/articles/323454

Food and Agriculture Organization (2011) Agricultural Labor. http://www.fao.org/3/i2490e/i2490e01b.pdf

Food and Agriculture Organization (2020). FAOSTAT. http://www.fao.org/faostat/en/#compare

Food and Agriculture Organization (2020). Nutritive Value of Roots and Tubers. http://www.fao.org/3/t0207e/T0207E04.htm

Food and Agriculture Organization of the United Nations. (2017). FAO cereal supply and demand brief. http://www.fao.org/worldfoodsituation/csdb/en/

Foundations of Western Culture (2020). Effects of Agriculture on the Industrial Revolution. http://foundations.uwgb.org/agriculture/

Fritz, H., Saïd, S., Renaud, P. et al. The effects of agricultural fields and human settlements on the use of rivers by wildlife in the mid-Zambezi valley, Zimbabwe. Landscape Ecol 18, 293–302 (2003). https://doi.org/10.1023/A:1024411711670

Fuller, D. Q., & Hildebrand, E. (2013). Domesticating plants in Africa. In The Oxford handbook of African archaeology. https://www.oxfordhandbooks.com/view/10.1093/oxfordhb/9780199569885.001.0001/oxfordhb-9780199569885-e-35

GuarinoL (2014).So how many crops feed the world anyway?. https://agro.biodiver.se/2014/03/so-how-many-crops-feed-the-world-anyway/

Gupta, Anil K. "Origin of Agriculture and Domestication of Plants and Animals Linked to Early Holocene Climate Amelioration." *Current Science*, vol. 87, no. 1, 2004, pp. 54–59. JSTOR, www.jstor.org/stable/24107979. Accessed 4 Aug. 2020.

Harris, K. A., & Kris-Etherton, P. M. (2010). Effects of whole grains on coronary heart disease risk. *Current atherosclerosis reports*, 12(6), 368-376.

Harvard health. Publishing (2015). Carbohydrates-Good or Bad for You?https://www.health.harvard.edu/diet-and-weight-loss/carbohydrates--good-or-bad-for-you

Henry, D. (1771). *The Complete English Farmer, Or, A Practical System of Husbandry...* F. Newbery.

History (2020). Industrial Revolution. https://www.history.com/topics/industrial-revolution/industrial-revolution https://www.scientificamerican.com/article/why-does-the-brain-need-s/

Hunter Course (2020). Amazing Hunter-Gatherer Societies. https://www.huntercourse.com/blog/2011/05/amazing-hunter-gatherer-societies-still-in-existence
IFASTAT (2020).Fertilizer Consumption.https://www.ifastat.org/databases/graph/1_1

Institute of Medicine (US) Committee on Social Security Cardiovascular Disability Criteria. Cardiovascular Disability: Updating the Social Security Listings. Washington (DC): National Academies Press (US); 2010. 7, Ischemic Heart Disease. Available from: https://www.ncbi.nlm.nih.gov/books/NBK209964/

International Fund for Agricultural Development, UNICEF, World Food Programme, & World Health Organization. (2019). The state of food security and nutrition in the World: Safeguarding against economic slowdowns and downturns. FAO.

Jennings, K (2019). 9 health benefits of eating whole grains. Published in Healthline. https://www.healthline.com/nutrition/9-benefits-of-whole-grains

JOHN YUDKIN, Evolutionary and Historical Changes in Dietary Carbohydrates, The American Journal of Clinical Nutrition, Volume 20, Issue 2, February 1967, Pages 108–115, https://doi.org/10.1093/ajcn/20.2.108

Khan Academy (2020). The Dawn of Agriculture. https://www. khanacademy.org/humanities/world-history/world-history-beginnings/birth-agriculture-neolithic-revolution/a/where-did-agriculture-come-from

Kuhn, S., Milasi, S., & Yoon, S. (2018). World employment social outlook: Trends 2018. Geneva: ILO.

Langlie, B. S., Mueller, N. G., Spengler, R. N., & Fritz, G. J. (2014). Agricultural origins from the ground up: archaeological approaches to plant domestication. American Journal of Botany, 101(10), 1601-1617.

Lowder, S. K., Skoet, J., & Singh, S. (2014). What do we really know about the number and distribution of farms and family farms in the world? Background paper for The State of Food and Agriculture 2014. http://www.fao.org/family-farming/detail/en/c/281544/

Manzella, D (2020). The Different Types of Carbohydrates. Verywell Health. https://www.verywellhealth.com/simple-and-complex-carbohydrates-and-diabetes-1087570

McKevith, B. (2004). Nutritional aspects of cereals. Nutrition Bulletin, 29(2), 111-142.

Morello, A (2017). Harvesting in Ancient Egypt. https://sciencing.com/harvesting-ancient-egypt-8915.html

Naidoo, U (2016). Nutritional Strategies to Ease Anxiety. Harvard Health Publishing. https://www.health.harvard.edu/blog/nutritional-strategies-to-ease-anxiety-201604139441

National geographic (2020). Evolution of diet. https://www.nationalgeographic.com/foodfeatures/evolution-of-diet/

National Osteoporosis Foundation(2020). Food and Your Bones-Osteoporosis Nutrition Guidelines. https://www.nof.org/patients/treatment/nutrition/

Non-GMO Projects (2020). GMO Facts. https://www.nongmoproject.org/gmo-facts/

Nugent, A. P. (2005). Health properties of resistant starch. Nutrition Bulletin, 30(1), 27-54. https://onlinelibrary.wiley.com/doi/full/10.1111/j.1467-3010.2005.00481.x

OECD-FAO (2016). Agricultural Outlook 2016-2025. http://www.fao.org/3/a-bo092e.pdf

Okay Africa (2019). What is Fufu? https://www.okayafrica.com/what-is-fufu-a-quick-guide-to-africas-staple-food/?rebelltitem=10#rebelltitem10

Pearson, K (2017). What are the Key Functions of Carbohydrates?. Healthline. https://www.healthline.com/nutrition/carbohydrate-functions#section4

Popcorn.org (2020). Different types of corn. https://www.pop-corn.org/Different-Types-of-Corn

Preston, J. C., & Sandve, S. R. (2013). Adaptation to seasonality and the winter freeze. Frontiers in Plant Science, 4, 167.https://www.frontiersin.org/articles/10.3389/fpls.2013.00167/full

Proctor,R. A. (1882). The Influence of Food on Civilization. The North American Review, 135(313), 547-563.https://www.jstor.org/stable/25118223?seq=1#metadata_info_tab_contents

Purugganan, M. D. (2019). Evolutionary insights into the nature of plant domestication. Current Biology, 29(14), R705-R714. https://www.sciencedirect.com/science/article/pii/S0960982219306232

Reez, E (2019). What Did Ancient Civilizations eat? An Archaeology Lab Experiment. Published in Science Friday. https://www.sciencefriday.com/educational-resources/what-did-ancient-civilizations-eat-an-archaeology-lab-experiment/

Roderuck, C. E., & Fox, H. (1987). Nutritional value of cereal grains. Nutritional Quality of Cereal Grains: Genetic and Agronomic Improvement, 28, 1-10.https://onlinelibrary.wiley.com/doi/full/10.1111/j.1467-3010.2004.00418.x

Rodriguez, D (2009). The Right Diet to Beat Tuberculosis. Everyday Health.https://www.everydayhealth.com/tuberculosis/the-right-diet-to-beat-tuberculosis.aspx

Scientific American (2012). Human Ancestors were Nearly all Vegetarians. https://blogs.scientificamerican.com/guest-blog/human-ancestors-were-nearly-all-vegetarians/

Scoditti, E., Massaro, M., Garbarino, S., & Toraldo, D. M.

(2019). Role of diet in chronic obstructive pulmonary disease prevention and treatment. Nutrients, 11(6), 1357. https://pubmed. ncbi.nlm.nih.gov/31208151/

Seto, K. C., Dhakal, S., Bigio, A., Blanco, H., Delgado, G. C., Dewar, D., ... & McMahon, J. (2014). Human settlements, infrastructure and spatial planning. https://www.ipcc.ch/site/assets/ uploads/2018/02/ipcc_wg3_ar5_chapter12.pdf

Sleep Foundation (2020). What are the Fats about Insomnia?. https://www.sleepfoundation.org/articles/what-are-facts-about-insomnia

Species domestication and human life. https://pages.vassar.edu/ realarchaeology/2018/09/30/the-domestication-of-species-and-the-effect-on-human-life/

Sudha, M. L., Soumya, C., & Prabhasankar, P. (2016). Use of dry-moist heat effects to improve the functionality, immunogenicity of whole wheat flour and its application in bread making. Journal of Cereal Science, 69, 313-320.

Swaminathan, N. (2008). Why Does the Brain Need So Much Power?

Sylvester-Bradley, R., & Folkes, B. F. (1976). Cereal grains: Their protein components and nutritional quality. Science Progress (1933-), 241-263. https://www.jstor.org/stable/i40135340

TBFacts.org (2020). Food and TB. https://tbfacts.org/food-tb/

The Editors of Encyclopedia Britannica (2020). Industrial revolution. https://www.britannica.com/event/Industrial-Revolution

The healthy People (2020). Food insecurity. https://www.healthypeople.gov/2020/topics-objectives/topic/social-determinants-health/interventions-resources/food-insecurity

Turcotte, M. M., Araki, H., Karp, D. S., Poveda, K., & Whitehead, S. R. (2017). The eco-evolutionary impacts of domestication and agricultural practices on wild species. Philosophical Transactions of the Royal Society B: Biological Sciences, 372(1712), 20160033. https://www.researchgate.net/publication/311444381_The_eco-evolutionary_impacts_of_domestication_and_agricultural_practices_on_wild_species

United Nations (2020). Population. https://www.un.org/en/sections/issues-depth/population/

University of Wisconsin-Madison (2018). Ancient farmers spared us from glaciers but profoundly changed Earth's climate. Science News. https://www.sciencedaily.com/releases/2018/09/180906141507.htm

US History (2020). Food, clothing and shelter. https://www.ushistory.org/civ/2b.asp

US History (2020). Hunter-Gatherers. https://www.history.com/topics/pre-history/hunter-gatherers
US History (2020). Stone Age. https://www.history.com/topics/pre-history/stone-age

US History (2020). Bronze Age. https://www.history.com/topics/pre-history/bronze-age?li_source=LI&li_medium=m2m-rcw-history

USDA (2020). Grain: World Markets and Trade. https://www.fas.usda.gov/data/grain-world-markets-and-trade

Van Acker, R., Rahman, M., & Cici, S. Z. H. (2017). Pros and cons of GMO crop farming. In Oxford Research Encyclopedia of

Environmental Science. https://ankarahee.meb.gov.tr/meb_iys_dosyalar/2020_01/22082932_MAKALE_3.pdf

Varraso, R., Chiuve, S. E., Fung, T. T., Barr, R. G., Hu, F. B., Willett, W. C., & Camargo, C. A. (2015). Alternate Healthy Eating Index 2010 and risk of chronic obstructive pulmonary disease among US women and men: prospective study. bmj, 350. https://www.bmj.com/content/350/bmj.h286

Wikipedia (2020). Timeline of food. https://en.wikipedia.org/wiki/Timeline_of_food

World Health Organization (2020). Diarrhoeal Disease. https://www.who.int/news-room/fact-sheets/detail/diarrhoeal-disease

World Health Organizations (2020). Tuberculosis. https://www.who.int/news-room/fact-sheets/detail/tuberculosis

Wu, H., Flint, A. J., Qi, Q., Van Dam, R. M., Sampson, L. A., Rimm, E. B., ... & Sun, Q. (2015). Association between dietary whole grain intake and risk of mortality: two large prospective studies in US men and women. JAMA internal medicine, 175(3), 373-384. https://pubmed.ncbi.nlm.nih.gov/25559238/

NOTES

CHAPTER EIGHT: STAPLES AS PART OF OUR HEALTHY DIET TODAY

1. Wu, H., Flint, A. J., Qi, Q., van Dam, R. M., Sampson, L. A., Rimm, E. B., Holmes, M. D., Willett, W. C., Hu, F. B., & Sun, Q. (2015). Association between dietary whole grain intake and risk of mortality: two large prospective studies in US men and women. JAMA internal medicine, 175(3), 373–384. https://doi.org/10.1001/jamainternmed.2014.6283

CHAPTER NINE: HOW STAPLES HELP OR HINDER AILMENTS AND DISEASES

1. BMJ-British Medical Journal. (2015, February 3). Healthy diet linked to lower risk of chronic lung disease. ScienceDaily. Retrieved September 23, 2020 from www.sciencedaily.com/releases/2015/02/150203190217.htm

www.ingramcontent.com/pod-product-compliance
Lightning Source LLC
Chambersburg PA
CBHW021330060726
47591CB00006B/1959